# NEW YOU

## DISCOVERING THE

# MAGIC PILL

## FOR HEALTH & HAPPINESS

I0099900

# GERALD L. KOSTECKA

## HYDRATION EXPERT & CERTIFIED
## NUTRITIONAL THERAPIST

*"Let thy food be thy medicine and thy medicine be thy food."*

**Hippocrates**
*Regarded as the father of modern medicine*

*"The food you eat can be either the safest and most powerful form of medicine or the slowest form of poison."*

**Ann Wigmore**
*Holistic health practitioner, naturopath and raw food advocate*

*"The groundwork of all happiness is health."*

**Leigh Hunt**
*19th-century English poet and writer*

*"Every living cell in your body is made from the food you eat. If you consistently eat junk food then you'll have a junk body."*

**Jeanette Jenkins**
*American fitness trainer and author*

NOTES:_____
_____

# MESSAGE FROM GERALD KOSTECKA

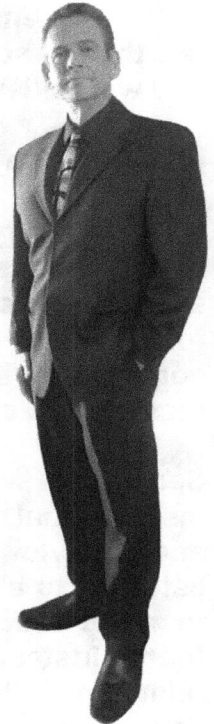

Congratulations on your commitment to improving your health! While making positive changes to your lifestyle can be challenging, it can also become the most rewarding journey of your life!

Remember that you are in control of your own health and well-being, and every small step you take towards better lifestyle choices add up over time. Every journey in life takes a first step and you've taken it! Be proud of yourself!

Don't get discouraged if you don't see immediate results or if you face setbacks along the way. It's important to be kind to yourself and focus on progress, rather than perfection. Every choice you make towards a healthy lifestyle is another step in the right direction, so take it step-by-step, day-by-day.

Remember to also seek and accept support from friends, family, or a healthcare professional as needed. You don't have to go through this journey alone.

Keep up the great work and keep striving towards your goals. You are capable of achieving them, and your efforts will pay off in the long run.

I believe in you and know you can accomplish what you set out to do and I am excited and honored to be part of your life-changing journey!

NOTES:_____
_____

# INTRODUCTION

Before we embark on this journey, I'd like to address a few things, so you'll know what to expect from this book and will understand how to get the most out of it.

First, you may have noticed that I use a larger font than most books. When I wrote my first alkaline ionized water industry book, *Ride The Wave*, I decided to use a larger font, as it made reading the text easier for me. As such, it would make it easier for others. The larger, bold font format is now my preferred approach when it comes to writing a book. I hope the larger font makes reading this easier for you too!

Second, I write the way I speak. I've read many instructional and informational books over the years and I never cared for the ones which remind me of listening to a lecture. I prefer conversational writing, so to make reading feel more like a friendly chat with a friend, instead of lessons from a stuffy instructor. Being relatable makes new information easier to digest and comprehend.

Third, I don't like using very technical sounding vocabulary. I'm not trying to impress you with all the flowery health related terms and words that I know. Is it really helpful to use unnecessary jargon to make myself sound more informed? I think not. I use normal, everyday words. For example, I may reference the color of pee as an indicator of hydration levels. Of course I know that pee is called urine, but why not write like most people actually speak? I mean, when was the last time you said, "Please excuse me, I must go urinate..."? Probably NEVER!! But I bet you've said the words, "Uh oh, I gotta pee!", at least once in your life. So expect easy to understand word usage in this book.

4

In order to get the most out of this book, it is extremely important to make a few decisions first. These are decisions that only you can make and that only you will know if you are actually following. Like a New Year's resolution, for it to work YOU must be the one to make it work!

The first task is to decide what is truly important to you. The title of this book includes the words "Health & Happiness", so it may be safe to assume that one or both of those things are important to you, but sometimes our actions do not correspond with what we say we want. We live in an age where we face more outside influences than ever before. These outside influences are typically bombarding us with what others want or expect us to be, despite what we want for ourselves. It can be overwhelming to figure out who we really are or what we really want, which is why this is an important part of the process.

If your health and happiness IS important to you, then you must decide to treat it like it is important and make it a priority. If you are unwilling or unable to do this, then you might as well put this book down and go about the rest of your day doing something else, as this book is not going to be able to help you. The ONLY people this book can possibly help are people who have decided that they have had enough and want to do what it will take to regain or maintain their health and their happiness!

This is one of those moments in life where what you do next can have a huge impact on your future. I hope you decide to make your health and happiness a priority! After all, in case no one has told you this today, YOU DESERVE TO BE BOTH HEALTHY AND HAPPY! And don't let ANYONE tell you otherwise!

NOTES:_____

_____

# GETTING STARTED RIGHT

My goal is to empower you with what I have learned over almost two decades and to allow you to quickly and efficiently learn what you will really need to successfully navigate your health journey.

One of the keys to getting started right is having the right attitude. While it is probably a bit cliché, attitude is everything! Good or bad, your attitude greatly influences all aspects of your life. In order to get the most out of this book, be sure that your attitude is properly aligned and prepared to make the most of it!

You are embarking on what could be the most important journey of your lifetime. While you are most likely filled with enthusiasm and excitement, you also need to be willing to learn, be open minded to new ideas and be determined to achieve your goals, no matter how many hurdles you may face. Along with all of this you need to have an above average, absolutely unbelievably positive attitude. With these things, you will be unstoppable. Without them, you will face a very rough ride!

I truly believe that having a positive attitude, coupled with the correct knowledge, can be the difference between a rough ride and an amazing journey. The attitude is ultimately up to you. All I can do is provide you with the correct knowledge, information, tips and suggestions that have worked for me and many other people.

So please, get started right and take this book seriously. Take notes and highlight sections that are of greatest importance to you. Treat this book like it can change your life for the better, because, if used correctly, it can!

NOTES:_____

_____

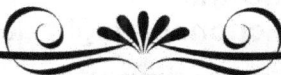

You are courageous!
It takes courage to pursue change.
It takes courage to face your own issues.
It takes courage to embark on a new journey.
You're doing all of these right now.
YOU ARE COURAGEOUS!

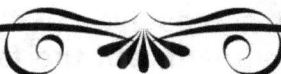

NOTES:_____

_____

# HEALTH – WHAT IS IT?

I think most people have a general idea of what health means, but let's define it, so we are all using the same definition. After all, the word "health" appears numerous times in this book. To be clear, this is my definition of health, so if I say something other than what is expected, understand that this is my viewpoint and not necessarily how a dictionary might define health.

I believe that the most important parts of the word health are the first four letters, which spells heal. In my opinion, health is the ability for the human body to heal. In addition, to me health is making lifestyle choices which allow or promote the ability for the body to heal itself. That would be my definition of living a "healthy" life. You see, the human body is absolutely incredible, as it is designed to be able to heal itself. The irony of an unhealthy body is that most of what makes it unhealthy has been self-induced, meaning we create most of our issues through our own lifestyle choices and actions.

I think another very important point is that health is ultimately each individual's personal responsibility. I know we live in a world where everyone is trying to duck responsibility, with a massive "…it's not my fault…" mentality running rampant, but the fact of the matter is that NO ONE should or will care more about your health than you, so you need to assume personal responsibility for your health, or you will lose it. That is a fact!

## *I'm becoming the me…*

## *…that I'm truly meant to be!*

8

NOTES:_____

_____

# ASSUMING PERSONAL RESPONSIBILITY

"It's not my fault!" Have you ever said this phrase? You, and just about every other person on this planet, including me, have probably said it at some point. I think it is basic human nature to not want to be the reason something doesn't work out correctly, but somehow assumption of personal responsibility has become almost taboo. It seems like more and more people are pointing the finger at others for the problems in their life.

Now this is not to say that things outside of our control do not happen, because they do. But it is important to be willing to assume personal responsibility for the things that are actually of our own doing. Placing blame on others is an easy way to duck having to assume responsibility, but it is not a healthy habit and one that each of us should try hard to break!

If you are going to make positive lifestyle changes, then you must be willing and able to confront the role you have played in your past decisions. I believe that one of the things currently causing a lot of societal problems is the lack of assumption of personal responsibility. There is a strong connection with the way individuals act and the way society responds to those actions, both good and bad. A lack of assuming personal responsibility on a personal level can have a devastating ripple effect on society.

Personal responsibility is a cornerstone of a healthy and successful individual, which then reflects on society. It refers to the notion that each individual is accountable for their own actions and decisions. Assuming personal responsibility means taking ownership of one's life and the outcomes that result from their choices and behavior. In this section, we will explore why personal

NOTES:_____

_____

responsibility is so critical and how it impacts both the individual and society as a whole.

First and foremost, personal responsibility empowers individuals to take control of their lives and make positive changes. When people take responsibility for their actions, they have the power to learn from their mistakes and make better choices in the future. This self-reflection and self-awareness is essential for personal growth and development. Furthermore, assuming personal responsibility can also increase one's self-esteem and confidence, as they are no longer blaming outside forces for their shortcomings.

Moreover, personal responsibility helps to foster a sense of community and interconnectedness. When people take responsibility for their actions, they are less likely to engage in negative behavior that can harm others. This, in turn, creates a safer and more harmonious environment for everyone. Additionally, by assuming personal responsibility, individuals can contribute to the betterment of society as a whole. For example, people who take responsibility for their own health and wellness can reduce the burden on the healthcare system, allowing resources to be directed towards those in need.

Another important aspect of personal responsibility is that it promotes accountability and fairness. When people are held accountable for their actions, they are more likely to act in an ethical and responsible manner. This creates a level playing field, where everyone is held to the same standards and no one can escape the consequences of their actions. Furthermore, assuming personal responsibility helps to ensure that individuals are held accountable for their own mistakes and do not pass the blame onto others.

NOTES:_____

_____

Even though it may be difficult or even uncomfortable to force yourself to assume personal responsibility for your own actions, it is imperative for personal growth and healthy societal development. It's time to stop the blame game!

When you start to assume personal responsibility, you will find that you will grow as a person. The mistakes in our lives are what give us the opportunity to grow, so do not shun these unfortunate events, embrace the chance to learn from them. The only way you can do that is to actually face the problem, not blame others or pretend it doesn't exist.

Reading this book is actually an excellent example of assuming personal responsibility! The majority of people who pick up a book called "New You" probably are not real happy with the old them, which is why they made the decision to pick up the book and read through the pages. This simple action is a clear assumption of responsibility and your willingness to change things that you have the power to change. The choices you've made in the past, no matter how self-destructive they may have been, are insignificant, as long as you learned from them and made changes to avoid them from happening again.

Things happen in life that put you in the right place at the right time. No matter what led up to your reading this book, you have assumed personal responsibility and you should be proud of yourself for taking this difficult step.

I'm not sure what circumstances brought you right here, right now; but I'm glad you made the decision to be right here, right now and I'm honored to be part of your life-changing journey! The journey of a thousand miles starts with a single step, so you are on your way!

11

NOTES:_____

_____

*Your life will be whatever you focus on…*

*That's what creates your life…*

*What you look at, look to, what you imagine…*

*These are the things you will create in your life.*

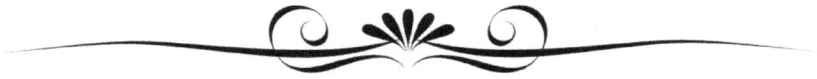

*Not happy with your life?*

*Don't focus on a new life…*

*Focus on a New You!*

12

NOTES:_____

_____

# GOAL SETTING

In this section we are going to discuss goal setting, but I want you to wait until you finish this book before you actually set any concrete health or weight loss goals. It will be more helpful for you to wait until you are armed with more knowledge to accomplish your goals than to set your goals prematurely.

For most people, a goal is a general idea instead of a specific destination. It is a poorly thought out wish, instead of a concrete direction. Saying that you want to lose a bunch of weight or get healthy, these are not goals, these are really nothing more than wishes, and unless you have a genie in a bottle, wishes don't really amount to very much. Without actual goals, you don't know what actions are necessary to turn them from wishes into reality.

In many of my business trainings I discuss SMART goals, which can apply to any type of goal setting, not just business. SMART goals are a popular framework for setting specific, measurable, achievable, relevant, and time-bound goals.

SMART stands for:

1. Specific: Clearly define what you want to accomplish.

2. Measurable: Make sure your goal can be quantified or tracked in some way.

3. Attainable: Make sure your goal is realistic and within reach.

4. Relevant: Ensure your goal aligns with your values and priorities.

5. Timeframe: Set a deadline for achieving your goal to provide motivation and a sense of urgency.

13

NOTES:_____

_____

Using the SMART framework can help you set effective and achievable goals that are more likely to lead to success. By focusing on each of the five elements, you can ensure that your goals are well-defined, attainable, and meaningful, giving you a roadmap for reaching your desired outcome.

When you identify goals that are most important to you, you begin to figure out ways you can make them come true. You develop the attitudes, abilities and skills to reach them. You begin seeing previously overlooked opportunities to bring yourself closer to the achievement of your goals.

You can attain almost any goal you set when you plan your steps wisely and establish a time frame that allows you to carry out those steps. Goals that may have seemed far away and out of reach eventually move closer and become attainable, not because your goals shrink, but because you grow and expand to match them.

Improving your health and losing weight are common goals for many people, but it can be challenging, so start SMART! Setting clear and achievable goals is a powerful tool that can help you stay on track and make real progress towards both improved health and weight loss. Here are some tips for setting effective goals for improved health and weight loss.

1.  Identify Your Priorities: Start by identifying the areas of your health and weight that are most important to you. Focus on one or two areas at a time and make these your top priorities.

2.  Be Specific: Specify exactly what you want to achieve and set a deadline. For example, instead of saying "I want to be healthier and lose weight," try saying "I want to exercise for 30 minutes a day, five

NOTES:_____

_____

days a week, and lose 10 pounds in the next three months."

3. **Make it Attainable:** Set realistic and attainable goals that are within your reach. This will help you stay motivated and avoid frustration. Start small and build on your progress over time. Your goal is probably realistic if you truly believe that it can be accomplished. Additional ways to know if your goal is realistic is to determine if you have accomplished anything similar in the past or ask yourself what conditions would have to exist to accomplish this goal.

4. **Set a Timeframe:** Goals cannot remain open ended, there must be a specific time to the goals you are setting. With no timeframe tied to your goals there's no sense of urgency. If you want to lose 10 pounds, when do you want to lose it by? "Someday?" That won't work. If you anchor it within a specific timeframe, "by the first day of summer", then you've set your unconscious mind into motion to begin working on the goal.

5. **Create a Plan:** Create a plan that outlines the steps you will take to reach your goals. This may include changes to your diet, exercise routine and daily habits. Make sure your plan is practical and achievable, and consider seeking the help of a professional, such as a registered dietitian or a personal trainer, to ensure you're on the right track.

6. **Track Your Progress:** Keeping track of your progress is important for motivation and accountability. Use a food diary, a weight loss tracker, and a fitness tracker or any other method that works best for you to monitor your progress. Celebrate your successes and acknowledge any setbacks, and adjust your plan as needed.

15

NOTES:_____

_____

7. **Be Positive:** A positive attitude is essential for success. Focus on what you can achieve, not what you can't. Celebrate your successes and don't be too hard on yourself if you encounter obstacles along the way.

8. **Revisit Your Goals:** Regularly revisit your goals to ensure they are still relevant and achievable. You may need to adjust your goals or timeline as you progress, and that's okay. The most important thing is to stay committed to your journey and keep moving forward.

Don't let your goals sit in your head; when setting your goals you have to write them down on paper. This is very important! Until a goal is written on paper, it is just a notion, an intangible, fleeting idea. Putting your goals on paper makes them real, it gives the notion substance, and it goes from simply an idea or thought, to something that actually exists! You can see it on the page. It becomes real. Remember, these are YOUR goals; they are not some kind of law. If you do not achieve a goal by a certain time, it's okay. Just revisit them and adjust accordingly.

Tell friends and family about your goals. By expressing your goals to them, you now have others holding you accountable for your actions. A little reminder from those you care about can be the thing that keeps you on track to completing your goal. So, when you reach the end of this book, that's when I suggest you set your goals. Be sure to reference back to this section when that times comes, so you can refresh your memory about this important topic and so you can be sure that the goals you set are just like you, SMART!

NOTES:_____

_____

# WHO AM I?

I always chuckle a little when I read a book and there is a section about the author. If it were accurately titled, to fit the needs of the reader, it would more appropriately be called, "Why should you consider listening to anything I have to say?" This is especially true for a self-help book. Let's be real, most readers did not pick up this book to learn about my life, they picked it up to see how this book can help them. But parts of my life are what inspired some of the results I've achieved. I also feel it is important for you to know my background, to understand who I am, because some of my experiences may be relatable to your own.

I'm an average person with above average hopes and aspirations. I did not come from a wealthy family and have had both my ups and downs. Some of the ups were incredibly high, like appearing on several nationally televised talks shows. Some of the downs were unfortunately very low, like being homeless and living in the back of a car for six months! I've had many accomplishments in life, but they were earned, not given to me, so I think I am a good example of what a person can do when they set their mind to something. As a result, I actually like helping others. Heck, I suffer from a "hero" complex, meaning that I am always mindful of others who are in distress, ready to save the day!

I have no problem admitting the poor decisions I've made in life. I have tried hard to recognize the lessons I should learn from my many experiences. Even the worst things in my life have taught me valuable lessons!

I believe that who we are today is the result of every experience we have ever had. This is one of the main reasons I refuse to accept a one-size-fits-all approach to

17

NOTES:_____

_____

anything in life. We are all different, but we may share similar experiences and when we overcome the challenges we are faced with, it can serve as inspiration for others who have also had similar experiences. In this section of the book, I am going to divulge some less than flattering things about myself. Things that I am not particularly proud of, but that I realize were instrumental for me to become the person I am today. Someone I am very happy to be!

I mention this to remind you that your past does not have to dictate your future, nor does it define you. If I believed what I've experienced would decide who I am, then I should probably be in prison or dead by now. Instead, I learned to overcome the negative situations, move past my own misgivings and recognize the value in even the worst things I've experienced. We can become whoever we want to be, no matter what we've gone through!

So when you look in the mirror or step on a scale and you're not happy with what you see, IT'S OKAY!! That is simply the person you are today, not the person you have to be forever. That is the beauty of this life. If we do not like who we are today, we can choose to change. We can take back control and achieve whatever our heart desires...we just have to decide to do it. Not just think about doing it, ACTUALLY do it! I made that decision long, long ago and I'm excited to share with you how I did it and the amazing results I've had since. I'm also excited that you chose to pick up this book, as that choice has the potential to help you as you embark on this new chapter of your story!

This book is simply me trying to help others with lessons I have learned about health, happiness and a bit of hydration. This even applies to the pictures I decided

NOTES:_____

_____

to include in the book. I did not run out to get professional pictures taken to try to impress anyone; in fact, all of the pictures you'll see included in this book are pictures from my real life, not some carefully constructed façade intended to create a specific reaction from the reader. I am one of those, "what you see is what you get" kind of people!

Before I dive into my past, I would like to discuss my health related experience and qualifications. I think these are important, since this book is about health. It's important to know that the person writing this book actually has experience in this area!

I have been in the alkaline ionized water and the health & wellness industry since 2007. I've done extensive research into the connection between proper hydration and good health, as well as many other aspects of health, including proper nutrition. I've written two alkaline ionized water industry books and written and published magazines and brochures about the alkaline water industry. I've also helped produce educational videos which are used by the entire industry to this day.

Before entering the alkaline ionized water industry, I had some work experience with health & wellness, as well as being very active when I was young. But discovering this unique water was quite literally a life saver for me and my family and has resulted in me not only becoming a sought after expert in the alkaline ionized water industry, but it also inspired my ongoing pursuit of knowledge and education regarding health.

This amazing water changed the entire direction of my life, which is why I refer back to it throughout this book. It became my gateway to wanting to know more about this thing we call health!

19

NOTES:_____

_____

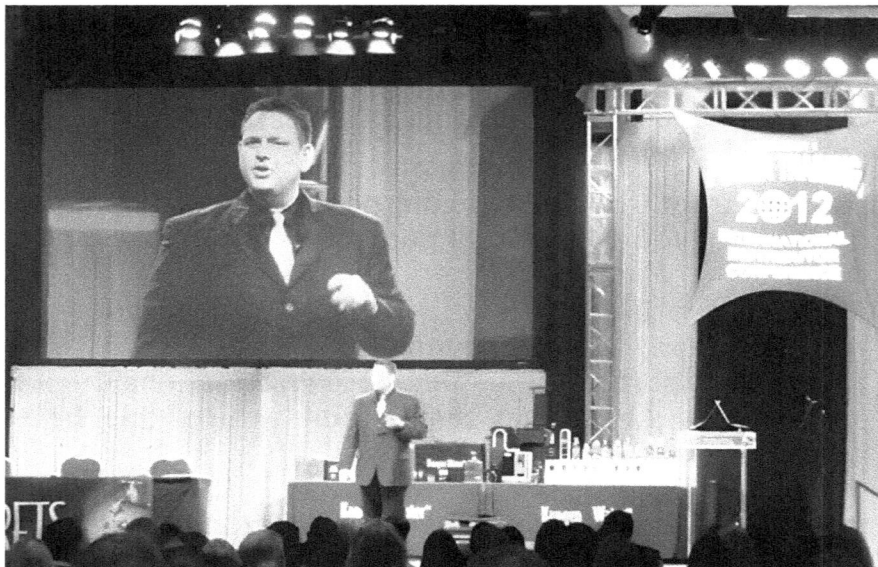

Prior to my involvement in the health & wellness industry, I was a writer, trainer and public speaker, which helped me immensely. Since starting in 2007, I have conducted hundreds of live seminars and have helped organize and been a keynote speaker at some of the biggest events in the alkaline ionized water industry.

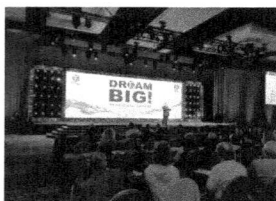

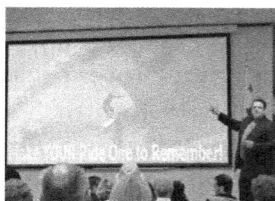

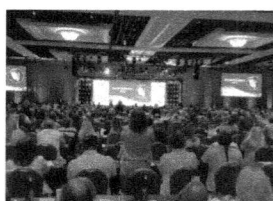

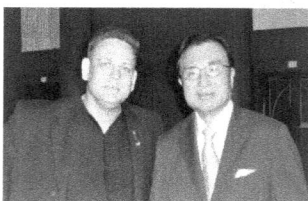

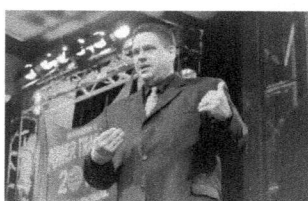

The pictures above are from some of the many events where I spoke. I've been a keynote speaker at numerous training events all over the United States, with as many as 4000 attendees.

20

NOTES:_____

_____

Not only have I learned a lot since becoming part of the health & wellness industry, but I've also had the unique opportunity to meet, talk to and work with people from all walks of life, including professional athletes, movie stars, singers, Gold Medal Olympians, social media influencers, health gurus, successful businesspeople and more. It has also allowed me to travel to amazing places around the world. I've even been recognized with awards for my achievements in the industry.

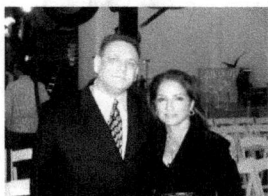

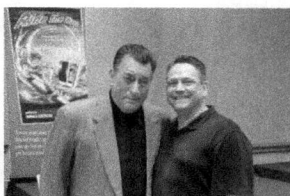

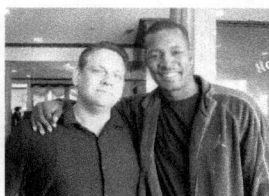

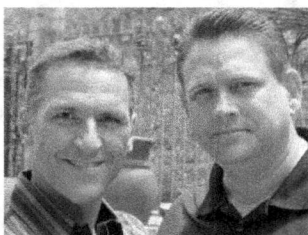

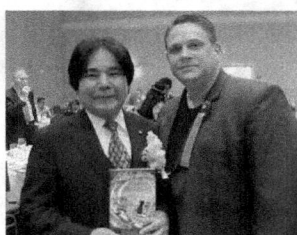

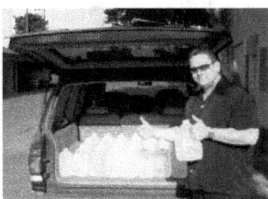

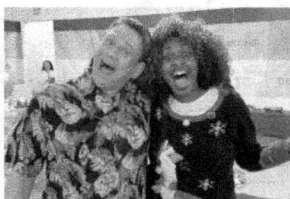

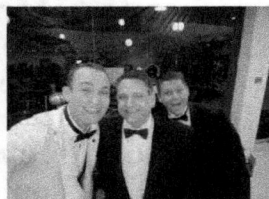

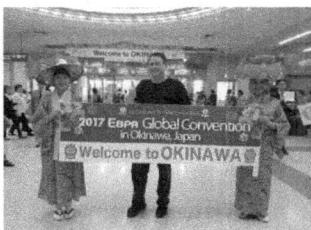

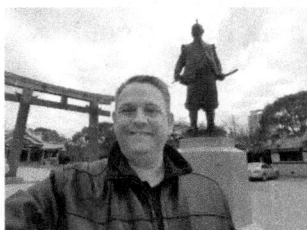

NOTES:_____

_____

My experiences and knowledge about health and wellness have opened many doors for me. I've been interviewed on television shows, news reports, radio broadcasts and in educational videos, which are used in the alkaline ionized water industry to this day.

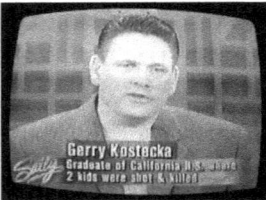

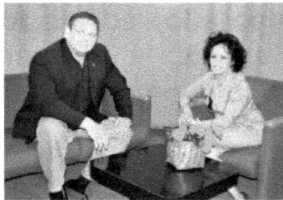

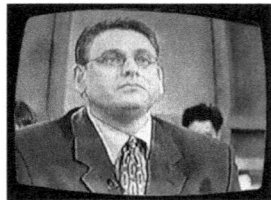

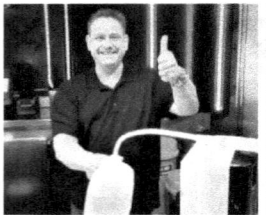

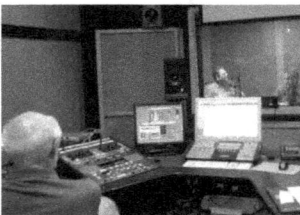

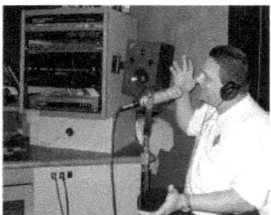

In addition to the books I've written, I've also written hundreds of health related articles, which have appeared online and in print. In 2018 I decided to expand my health & wellness knowledge and enrolled in a course to become a Certified Nutritional Therapist. I successfully completed the course and received my professional diploma in 2019. I'm proud to say that I have personally helped thousands of families around the world discover improved health through proper hydration and nutrition. In addition to my professional experience, I've also had my own journey of improved health and now I want to share what I've learned with you!

These are just a few of the reasons I feel you should consider listening to what I have to say. Now here is a little about the life that brought me to where I am today.

NOTES:_____

_____

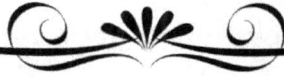

Life is actually pretty simple…
If you look for problems, you will find problems.
If you look for solutions, you will find solutions.
If you ignore health, you will become unhealthy.
If you improve health, you will become healthy.
Lesson: look for solutions and improve health.
It's really that simple!

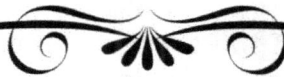

NOTES:_____

_____

# HOW MY LIFE INSPIRED THIS BOOK

From the day I was born I was faced with challenges. I was born with a condition called Pectus Excavatum, which causes a concave sternum. As a newborn, if you put a finger on the most sunken part of the middle of my chest, you could actually feel my spinal cord. The doctors told my mother I would be lucky to live to a year or two; that as I grew, my inverted chest bone would most likely pierce my heart and kill me. They made things even worse by telling my mother there would be nothing they could do about it. So for the first few years of my life, there was a constant fear that one day I would just fall over and die.

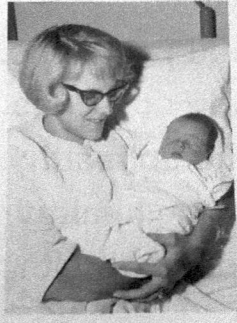

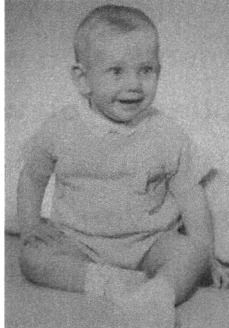

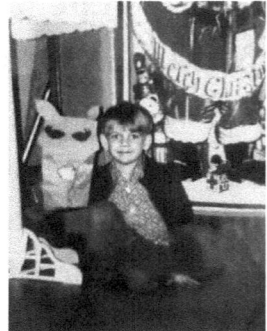

But somehow I defied the odds and grew from infant, to a toddler, to an energetic and active child. However, when I was sixteen months old my baby sister, who was three months old at the time, did pass away. This was more than my parents could handle and led to their divorce. My biological father was never in my life during my childhood, so my mother raised me and my older sister on her own.

In order to ensure that she would have steady employment and medical benefits for me and my sister my mother joined the Navy and when I was five we

24

NOTES:_____

_____

moved to San Diego, CA. Back in the mid 1970s life for an enlisted woman who was divorced with two kids wasn't easy, but we managed, living in Navy housing for the majority of my pre-teen childhood.

I was short and skinny, but had loads of energy, so much so that I was often seen as a disruption in school. Because of my size, I was picked on by bullies, which created a disdain for those who bully others, something which has stuck with me all my life. As a result of my excess energy I was branded a bit of a "problem child", with comments like "won't sit still", "doesn't pay attention" and "talks excessively" on almost every report card.

I was very physical and taught myself how to do gymnastics and became strong and was fast...very fast. In fifth grade I participated in the Presidential Physical Fitness tests and ended up being the fastest kid in the entire school. In sixth grade my teacher, Mrs. Reich, recognized something in me that no other adult must have ever seen. Against the wishes of the school principle, she recommended that I help conduct the weekly Friday assembly.

I became a bit more focused as I started public speaking in front of about 750 students, teachers and parents each week and ended up running and being elected the President of Student Council. This was my first taste of public speaking and being rewarded by people outside of my family for the hard work I was doing. I was very intelligent and returned borderline genius level scores on a school given I.Q. test, but never really stood out academically.

Things took a major turn for the worse for me when my mother remarried when I was thirteen years old. There

25

NOTES:_____

_____

were major problems between me and my stepfather, problems which would have life-altering results. My stepfather and mother were both in the Navy and shortly after their marriage our new family was stationed overseas. We moved to Subic Bay, Philippines for two years. After that we returned to the San Diego area and things between me and my stepfather became even worse.

The next several years were a roller-coaster ride of emotions and confusion. I was thrust into a world of high-priced psychiatrists, locked psychiatric hospitals, juvenile detention facilities and out-of-state residential placement. After over a year and a half of being shuffled back and forth to different placements, I returned to the home of my mother and stepfather. With about six months before my 18th birthday, I moved out and started supporting myself.

There I was, seventeen and a half years old, living on my own, working a job and trying to finish high school. It was at this time I also started experimenting with illegal drugs, specifically methamphetamine. Circumstances beyond my control forced me to return to my parent's home about two months later and a final altercation with my stepfather made me pack my bags and leave. I was picked up by the police the next day as a runaway and was taken to Juvenile Hall. I stayed there for a month and was then accepted into the East County Gatehouse, a group home for displaced youth. My stay would last until the day of my 18th birthday.

The three years since returning back from the Philippines had been very difficult for me. My first night at the Gatehouse was truly eye opening for me and I literally had a life-changing epiphany. I arrived late and the other residents were all asleep. The staff member

NOTES:_____
_____

on duty, David, welcomed me and asked me to explain what brought me to their facility.

I spent the next few hours detailing all of the things I had endured over the years; from childhood bullies, to my stepfather, to my drug use and the years bouncing around the "system". I was articulate, detailed and passionate as I recounted all the terrible things that had happened to me and the scoundrels who had wronged me. I sat back, giving a smile of relief; proud of myself for surviving all of the things I had been subjected to and being able to share these very personal and private thoughts and feelings so eloquently.

After the several hours of respectfully listening to me drone on about my past, David let me finish and simply said, "Wow, you make a lot of excuses don't you!" I was flabbergasted! Had he not heard a word I said? Was he not listening to me at all? How could THIS be his response to the outpouring of my soul? Confused, I asked him a very direct question, "Why would you say that?"

His answer still echoes in my mind, helping me deal with things to this day. "Well, I listened to everything you said and from what I heard, you place blame on your situation on everyone except for yourself. Do you really want to give all the people you spoke about that much power over the outcome of your life?"

No one had ever put it like that to me. That by placing blame on everyone else, I was allowing them to greatly impact my self-worth, my attitudes, my abilities, even the direction of my future. I'm not sure why his short response had such a profound impact on me, but those poignant words were exactly what I needed to hear and they really changed my life!

27

NOTES:_____

_____

Remember one of the first sections of this book about personal responsibility? Well, now you know why I included that section and why I feel it is so important. I am living proof that assuming personal responsibility can completely change your life! That doesn't mean I haven't made my share of bad choices, because I have, but I assumed responsibility for those choices and have learned from my mistakes!

I had allowed my young life to spiral out of control and I now faced the harsh reality of being an adult in just a few short months. In that moment I decided to stop blaming the world for my woes, changed my outlook and my direction. My first major decision was that I wanted to earn my high school diploma.

At that time I should have been in my senior year; however, my school records only showed me completing half my sophomore year, as most of my school transcripts had been lost during all the moves over the previous several years.

To graduate I would need to complete two and a half years of school work in less than three months! I wasn't going to accept excuses, especially from myself, and I decided when I want something, I'll put my nose to the grind stone, do the work and get it done! So I made a commitment to myself to do what needed to be done.

I spent each day completing between 5 and 10 assignments per day, per subject, while also having a job with a roofing company. It was hard work, but that work, and emotional support from the Gatehouse staff, paid off for me. I completed all of the required assignments in less than three months and was presented with a high school diploma on my 18th birthday in a formal ceremony on the front lawn of the

NOTES:_____

_____

Gatehouse. The staff even rented a cap and gown and bought a graduation cake for me, the single graduate of my Class of 1986.

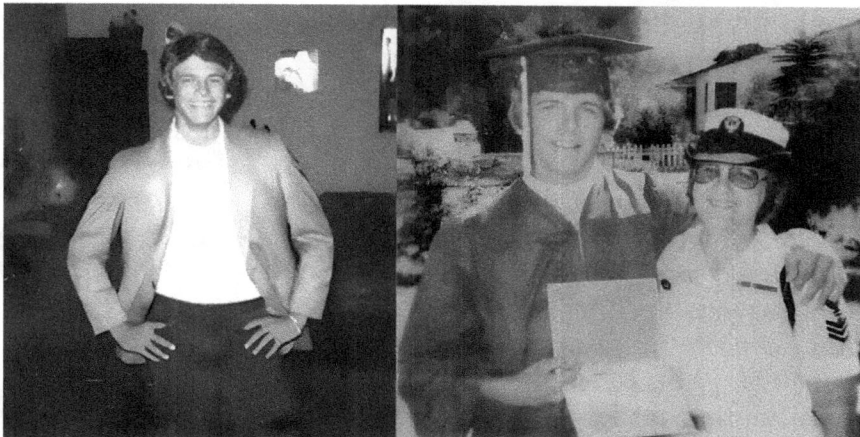

I was suddenly an adult and thrust into a world for which I wasn't really prepared. Unfortunately, the reality of my situation got the best of me and a lack of direction and newfound freedom took me back into a world of drug use and additional antisocial behavior. In fact, I spent the next few years in this world, until Nicholas, the first of my three children, was born. I started working and stopped using drugs.

My relationship with my son's mother was rocky at best and it deteriorated even more, but not before she became pregnant with my second child. Our relationship was over before my daughter, Khailey, was even born. My children stayed mostly with their mother for the first few years and I fell back into some of my bad habits, something that can happen to even the best of us! I was again using meth, being very irresponsible and I started drinking heavily, which eventually led to a DUI. This became one more of those "wakeup calls" for me and helped point me in a better direction.

29

I finally started to act more responsibly by maintaining steady employment and became the primary caregiver for my children. I worked with developmentally disabled at a place called the Home of Guiding Hands as a Residential Service Technician. This was my first exposure to medical training.

As part of the job's requirements, I learned Advanced First Aid and became CPR Certified. I also took in-service courses like Management of Assaultive Behavior, which prepares you for behavioral challenges, including physical and verbal outbursts, self-injury, aggression, and property destruction. This was the job that created the beginning foundations for greater learning about health and helped develop my appreciation and desire to help others.

I started writing again, which had been a way to express my feelings when I was a teenager. I focused attention on a poem I had written for creative writing credits while at the Gatehouse. The poem was the birthplace of the Dream Dragon. My creative juices started flowing again and I began writing Dream Dragon stories.

A new job had me traveling to Orange County, CA where I met a beautiful young lady named Susan. She would become my wife, mother of my third child and my inspiration to become something great. I knew that I needed to move from where I was. There were too many opportunities to fall back into those bad habits again and I really did not want that to happen. I relocated to Orange County and married Susan about a year later. My third child, Nathaniel, soon joined us. This is when I finally decided to take my life back. I cleaned up my act and made the decision to be fully committed to my family and my dreams. In fact, as of the writing of this book, I have been sober from meth for nearly 30 years!

30

NOTES:_____

_____

Several opportunities allowed me to grow professionally, including professional training as a public speaker and business seminar presenter. I excelled and considered the pursuit of my dream of becoming a published writer. In 1999, I turned this dream into a reality by forming Dragon Tales Publishing, LLC. Writing under the pen name Nyle Steck, I published my first children's picture book, *Dreamtime Friend*, which featured the Dream Dragon, a character I created in a poem I wrote while working towards my high school diploma.

As a result of my children's book project I have been interviewed for print articles, on talk radio shows and nationally televised television talk shows. I appeared on the Sally Jessy Raphael Show, Protecting America's Kids: Who's To Blame, where I addressed the parental role regarding student involved school shootings. I also appeared on the Rob Nelson Show, The New Sexual Revolution: Teen & Pre-Teen Sex in America, where I discussed parental responsibility regarding teen and pre-teen sex education. I started gaining experience in areas I never would have expected or thought possible. Unfortunately, circumstances beyond my control forced me to put my Dream Dragon efforts on hold, but I always believed that someday, when the time was right, the Dream Dragon would once again take flight.

I spent the next few years working hard to build a good life for my family. At times things got very tough, especially financially, but I had the love of my family, which was enough to motivate me to keep forging forward. My experiences had taught me some very valuable lessons, in both business and life and I was willing to work hard, which opened doors of opportunity for me, I just hadn't been able to find a place where I felt I really fit and could excel.

31

NOTES:_____

_____

I started doing sales of investment leads and I was very good at it. As a result, I started doing very well financially, better than I had ever done. This experience opened a door to an opportunity that allowed me to become the Director of Sales & Marketing for a marketing company. The main client was a telecommunications company. I worked for this company for roughly five years, until the company was dissolved at the end of 2006.

At the beginning of 2007 I was introduced to water ionizers and the alkaline ionized water industry by Daniel, who had been the Chairman of the marketing company. This is actually where this section of the book started. I have been working in this industry since then, but have also pursued some of my other interests.

As I became more financially successful, I also became active in the community and with charitable organizations, including working closely with Denise Brown of the Nicole Brown Charitable Foundation. I also served on the Board of Directors for several non-profit organizations, including as a board member of The Kids Cancer Connection and Vice-President of First Book. Over the next decade I worked hard and gained valuable life and business experience which would allow me to change my life and the life of my family.

Jump to the beginning of 2020, as the pandemic was just getting started, I could barely recognize the place the world had become. After seeing such a massive decline in society as a whole and seeing what was happening to our youth, I realized that the "right time" for the Dream Dragon was right now! I redesigned and re-released my original picture book and started writing again. I added a brand new group of characters, The Knights of Catcher's Table, to my Dreamland universe,

NOTES:_____

created a few coloring and activity books, made some t-shirt designs, had prototypes of a stuffed Dream Dragon and Sparks the Dragon plush toy made and assembled a team to produce and introduce the Dream Dragon animated series pilot, *Adventures In Dreamland: The Sour Case of the Candy Crops*. I had used my success in the alkaline ionized water industry to fund my life-long passion project. (www.thedreamdragon.com)

The Dream Dragon & The Dreamland Universe

In the next section we will continue into the craziness of 2020 so you can understand the rest of this story.

You may be wondering why I've included so much of my past in a book about creating a New You. I think it's important for you to know me, so you can see that the idea of a New You is realistic and possible. I know because my first New You success story was me! I've lived a real life, just like most other people.

I wasn't born into privilege, I've experienced just about every struggle in the book and I've had accomplishments and failures. I've had devastating heartbreak and I've experienced love to degrees I never thought possible. I've helped create life and I've had my share of loss. I've opened my life to you in the hopes that by sharing my past, I may be able to help you as you focus on a future with the New You!

33

# HOW THE PANDEMIC IMPROVED MY HEALTH

Before we proceed, I want to warn readers that I have included some pictures of what was happening in my life during this time and they may be hard for some to see, but sometimes in order to move forward in life, we have to face things, no matter how uncomfortable they may be. Some of these pictures may be hard to see. Heck, some were hard for me to revisit. Sometimes life can punch you square in the nose and I want you to know I've taken my share of punches! But healing cannot come until you face the problems that need to be healed!

Like most people around the world, I had no idea that 2020 was going to be the start of a series of life-changing events for me and my family. We lived in California during the majority of the pandemic and rules there were very strict, but I wanted to keep my family safe, so we took things seriously and hunkered down. My wife has a number of immune deficiencies, so we were careful even before the pandemic ever started. I was the main breadwinner of the family and I already worked from home, so it was pretty easy for us to adhere to lockdowns. In fact, my wife and son stayed home for over two years and I took care of anything that required leaving the house, like grocery shopping.

On a Friday in May of 2020 my brother-in-law, who was disabled and had been living with us for four years, suffered a brain aneurysm. My wife discovered him on the floor in his room. My son jumped into action and comforted him, while I was on the phone with 911. After what seemed like an eternity the EMT's arrived and he was taken to the hospital. He had a stroke about 10 years prior and doctors believed he had suffered

NOTES:_____

_____

another, more massive, stroke and they told us things did not look good for his recovery or even survival.

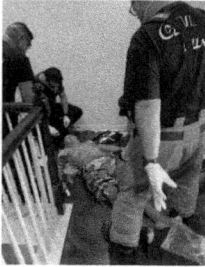

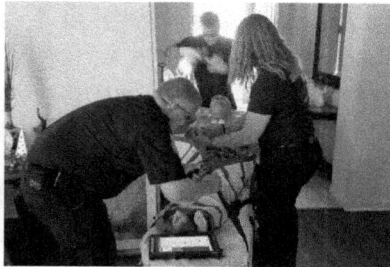

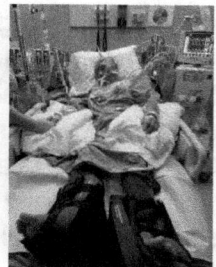

Like most people do in the event of a medical emergency, we reached out to family and friends to notify them. One of the people I tried to contact was Mike, one of my best friends of over thirty years. He was twenty years my senior and had become both a friend and father figure to me. Although we were not related, he was my family and over the years he had become a regular fixture during holidays, but had missed the last few as a result of a cancer issue.

Because of how chaotic things had been with my brother-in-law's hospitalization I didn't think much about it when I did not immediately hear back from him. But when things calmed down the next day, and I had still not heard back from him, I became concerned. I contacted law enforcement in his area to request a welfare check and they went out to his house.

The officer contacted me and said that everything looked fine, but I asked if his cars were in the driveway and when they said they were, I pleaded with them to gain entry. I told the officer he was in there and may need help. I received a call about twenty minutes later from the officer and was notified that he was found inside and that he was deceased. He had succumbed to the cancer.

35

NOTES:_____

_____

The hospitalization of my brother-in-law from a brain aneurysm and the discovery of my deceased best friend happened in less than twenty-four hours. As you can probably imagine, the stress level at that point was as high as it could be, at least that's what we thought at the time, but we were wrong. On Sunday, which was day three of this crazy situation, the hospital contacted us to tell us that the prognosis for my brother-in-law was not good and that we should probably prepare ourselves to say final goodbyes. At this point they still did not know that he had a brain aneurysm and still thought he had suffered a massive stroke.

My wife had been designated as the person to make the medical decisions on his behalf and the hospital was recommending that he be taken off life support, as they did not think he would recover. After a lot of soul searching the decision was made to take him off life support.

My brother-in-law had been a very independent person and we knew he would not want to be confined to a bed, being kept alive by a machine. We were all a wreck as we prepared ourselves for final goodbyes and scheduled to go to the hospital the next day. Keep in mind, this is five months into the pandemic, so protocols at the hospital were extensive and only two of us would be permitted to visit him at one time.

The next day my sister-in-law drove up from San Diego to go to the hospital with my wife and I so we could say goodbye. For some reason I had a weird feeling and I reached out to another friend who knew my friend Mike and asked him to swing by his place to make sure everything was secure.

NOTES:_____
_____

Twenty minutes before we were supposed to go to the hospital, my friend called me back to inform me that Mike's front door was wide open and that two people were going in and out, loading boxes into a truck parked outside. I lost it. The two people doing this were a relative of Mike's and someone Mike had considered a trusted friend. The police were called and they fled the scene. It was later discovered that they had broken in and were helping themselves to Mike's belongings. Then, after all that, we had to head to the hospital to basically send my brother-in-law to the Lord.

They say that when it rains it pours. Well, in that moment, it was pouring harder than I had ever experienced in my entire life. My heart was broken, my spirit was shattered and I was doing my best to keep it together for the sake of my wife and the rest of the family. We went to the hospital and my wife and sister-in-law went up to say their goodbyes, while I waited downstairs for my turn to say goodbye.

After about thirty minutes my wife came outside and said that her sister was convinced that their brother was responding to her. My wife figured it was more wishful thinking, and that any "response" was more likely involuntary, but I told her that I would go up and if he was responsive, I would make sure of it.

When I got to the hospital room my sister-in-law was adamant that he was responding. At first glance, he looked pretty bad and my gut told me that it was probably more wishful thinking than anything else. I came to the bedside and took my brother-in-law's hand into mine. "If you can hear me Don, I really need you to respond…squeeze my hand if you can hear me."

37

I waited a moment and felt a light squeeze. My heart jumped, but I did not want to rush to any conclusions, so I said it again, and, again, another light squeeze. This time I set his hand down onto the bed and said, "Don, if you can hear me, I need you to raise your left arm." His left arm rose off the bed about six inches and then returned to his side. After all the heartache of the previous four days, I was still not convinced, so I asked him to raise his arm again. Once again, his arm raised about six inches and then returned to the bed.

At this point I was elated and furious. Elated that he could hear us and was responding; furious that the hospital had said he was completely unresponsive and recommended that we come say goodbyes and essentially kill my brother-in-law. I told my sister-in-law to go down and tell my wife to come back up and that we were not taking him off life support. She went to get my wife and I kept talking to him.

I left the room and went to the elevators to meet my wife. When she came out of the elevator, I started explaining what was happening as we walked to his room. When we entered the room, my wife went to the bedside and I went to the foot of the bed. Suddenly, my brother-in-law opened his eyes, turned his head and looked right at my wife. She lost it with an outpouring of relief and just kept repeating, "I love you, Don!"

At that moment I realized that he knew our voices, but couldn't see our faces, because we were all wearing N-95 masks, and that he was probably very confused. I tore off my mask and started talking to him. I rushed out to get a nurse and then informed the hospital staff that there would be no goodbyes said that day! They did more tests the next day and discovered the brain aneurysm and finally started treating his actual

38

condition. Little did we know that the few days leading up to this day were going to create a domino effect that would drastically change our lives and the health of my whole family.

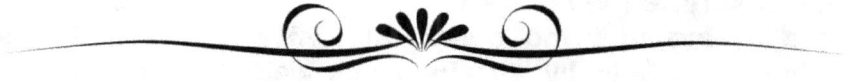

*Try to see something
good in everything.*

*Being positive is a choice!*

*In life your happiness depends on
the quality of your thoughts.*

*Never forget, being positive does
not mean you ignore the
negative, it means being able to
overcome the negative!*

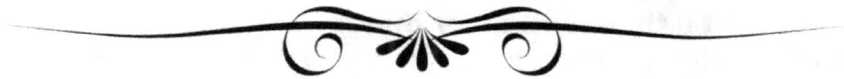

39

NOTES:_____

_____

# STRESS EATING TAKES A TOLL

After everything that had happened, my mother and sister, who only lived a few blocks from us, started bringing us food and homemade baked goods and we gladly gobbled it up. Our diet includes being gluten free and my mom and sis had become VERY good gluten free bakers, so we were happy to accept anything they were willing to bring over. Almost every meal I was eating was basically a train wreck waiting to happen. I was eating a pound of chicken tenders, along with a pound of french fries, followed by a third of a cake or a dozen cookies or 5 cupcakes!

Stress was taking its toll and my whole family was dealing with it by stress eating, which isn't actually dealing with it at all. All we were doing was making matters worse, but when your reality seems bleak it can be very difficult to recognize the bad things you're doing to yourself. It is a very unhealthy coping mechanism, mainly because it is not really coping; it is more of a temporary distraction that allows you to think less about the real issues. Facing these issues head on is more difficult, but much more productive and healthy!

I'm sure most people reading this can relate in some way to stress eating. Like I said, it is one of the easiest ways to deal with stress, but one of the worst for you. But, in the moment, I was not thinking about what the food I was eating was doing to me, I was just thinking about my recently deceased friend, the uncertainty of the ongoing pandemic, my hospitalized brother-in-law and about a thousand other things. All the stress eating was about to come to a head and life was about to completely change.

NOTES:_____

_____

# SPOUSAL INSPIRATION

A few weeks after my brother-in-law was hospitalized my wife and I were watching a few shows and she turned to me and said that she thought something was wrong. As I turned to look at her I immediately noticed that one of her eyes was completely crossed. At first I thought she was playing around, but I soon realized that this was no joke and that my wife was experiencing a major problem.

We thought this may be a temporary issue from all the stress, so we waited until the next day to see how she was doing. In the meantime, she started doing research into possible causes of this type of problem. We have never been the type of people who just run to a doctor's office if something seems off, in fact, since becoming part of the health and wellness industry nearly two decades ago, we had probably been to a doctor just a handful of times and those were for issues we felt we couldn't handle ourselves. We had always preferred to try to stay healthy by making better lifestyle choices and, for the most part this was effective, but the current situation was more than our bodies or minds could handle.

Her research was pointing at the possibility of her being diabetic, so when her eye issue continued the next day, we decided to go to the E.R. to have her checked out. We arrived at the E.R. and waited for my wife to be seen. Keep in mind this is back in 2020 at the height of the pandemic scare, with very little actual information being made available, so the mood was even more tense and uncomfortable than most E.R. visits.

We were also living in California, where things were being shut down to a degree that most other parts of the

NOTES:_____

_____

country never experienced. Even the trip to the E.R. was difficult, as the hospital was requiring very stringent rules for patients regarding N-95 facemasks and other protective gear. The global situation, our personal situation and the uncertainty of everything were unnerving, but my wife was having a serious issue and we needed to know exactly what was happening.

After several hours of waiting we were seen by a doctor and it was determined that whatever was happening wasn't life threatening, but to be safe, the doctor ordered bloodwork to be done. We waited for the results and were told that they thought my wife had become diabetic, as her A1C levels were elevated. When sugar enters your bloodstream, it attaches to hemoglobin, which is a protein in your red blood cells.

Everybody has some level of sugar attached to their hemoglobin, but people with higher blood sugar levels have more. The A1C test measures the percentage of your red blood cells that have sugar-coated hemoglobin. This test is the primary way to test if a person is diabetic. Based on her elevated levels, she was referred to our primary care physician for additional testing. She was deflated and almost defeated as a result of the confirmation of what she had deduced from her research, that she had developed diabetes.

The next few days were tough. She was depressed about the diabetes, as both of her parents had dealt with this issue and she feared she would be facing a lifetime of prescription dependency. To clarify, no one in our household was taking any prescription medications, and we still don't, so the thought of possibly needing medication for the rest of her life was eating at her. We were running around to doctor's appointments, eye specialist and to different labs for more bloodwork. It

42

NOTES:_____

_____

was mentality exhausting. She was still having the uncontrollable eye issue, so we got her an eyepatch to reduce the double vision issue.

I have always been kind of a jokester, feeling that even the tensest situation can be made easier with a little levity, and this was no exception. My wife was wearing an eyepatch, so naturally I started talking to her like a pirate! It brought a smile to her face, which is what I had hoped. Some may feel this would be inappropriate, but that's because you don't know us. Our dynamic is such that if I didn't do something stupid like that, she would have thought something was really wrong. And even if it was, with everything that was happening, I did not need her consumed by those kinds of thoughts. So for the next few days I was basically Jerry the Pirate! Arrrr!

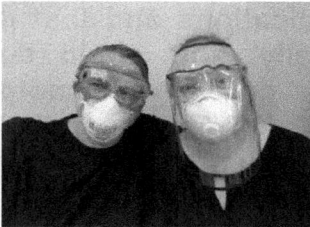

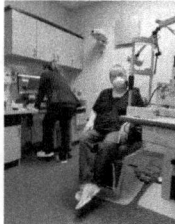

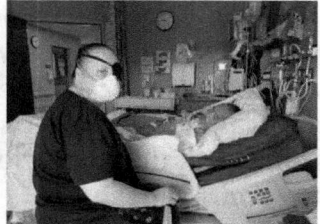

I think it is important to note that during all of this my brother-in-law was still in the hospital and we were on the phone with his doctors on a daily basis. He had undergone a surgery for the aneurysm and had been moved from the ICU. This was during the beginning of the pandemic, but we were being allowed to visit him, as we were not sure if he would stabilize or recover. Every day was difficult, but we persevered as much as we could while visiting my brother-in-law and going to my wife's medical appointments.

A few days after the trip to the E.R. my wife received a call from a nurse practitioner from our physician's

NOTES:_____
_____

office. He was calling to let her know that the bloodwork results had come in and what their office was going to recommend. My wife was told that her A1C levels were more than just "elevated", and that according to the lab results they were 10.6. For context, levels under 5.7 are considered normal and above 6.5 are considered diabetic, so hers were very high. She immediately started asking what she could do to deal with this naturally, as she knows the resilience of the body and that an issue like this, which wasn't genetic, could be handled without medication.

The next few minutes of the conversation were unfortunate and fortunate at the same time. She was told that she needed to start taking an oral diabetes medicine called Metformin immediately or there could be dire consequences. She explained that she did not want to become dependent on medications and that if told how to deal with this naturally, she would do whatever it took. Her request to be pointed in a more natural direction was met with what can only be called scare tactics, something that my family does not respond well to.

This phone call was happening on a Friday and she was told if she didn't start taking the medication that day, she would probably go blind or have a stroke over the weekend. Remember when I said this conversation was both unfortunate and fortunate at the same time? It was unfortunate that this healthcare representative was using scare tactics to try to get a patient to take medication, but it was fortunate because what he said was EXACTLY what my wife needed to hear to motivate her to never have to take any diabetes medicine.

I want to be clear that I am in no way recommending that a person not follow the advice or recommendations of

NOTES:_____

_____

their healthcare professional. Each situation is different and it is important that every person follow what they feel will be best for them, including exactly what your doctor recommends if you feel that is best. But in this situation, my wife had already devoted countless hours to researching different holistic and natural ways to reduce and even reverse her diabetes, so she wasn't happy with the obvious tactics being used to get her to do what they wanted.

She ended the call and immediately called the doctor's office back, to let them know that she never wanted that person to contact her again and that if that person did contact her again, we would be finding a new primary care physician. In hindsight that conversation was precisely what she needed to motivate her, so in the moment it was the last thing she WANTED to hear, but I believe that was what she NEEDED to hear.

That day became the start of a transformation that our own doctor's office wouldn't believe. We sat down as a family and talked about what would need to be done. At that time the conversation was centered around my wife, but the reality was that we all needed to make some changes, but we focused on her first.

One of the hardest parts of the changes my wife needed to implement had to do with her eating habits. Looking at her, you probably wouldn't believe that she is half Vietnamese. Her parents met in Vietnam when her father was stationed there while in the military. Rice had been a staple part of her mother's eating habits and it became a main part of her eating habits too and she loved it. Unfortunately, she discovered that rice, and most other starchy foods, are not recommended for people with diabetes.

45

NOTES:_____

_____

True to her word that she would do what was necessary to improve her current health condition, that day she stopped eating rice. Her eating habits were going to have to undergo some additional changes, especially because we had been eating so poorly since all the craziness of our situation had started. She was determined to fix the problem that she had created and I was ready to help her.

In addition to changes to her eating habits, she also implemented intermittent fasting to her daily routine. Her research had uncovered potential benefits from this practice, so she decided to give it a try. She also started a new daily exercise regimen. We had a stationary bike that had been collecting dust, so she dusted it off and started riding every day. At first she could only handle about ten minutes on the bike, but by the time we were getting ready to move a few years later she had built up to almost an hour and a half!

I was anxious to help her, although at that time I wasn't really thinking about what that was really going to mean. I figured that I would cook her dinners to make things easier. When I was younger I had worked in a restaurant as a cook and had always enjoyed cooking, so I put on my apron and started making dinners for my wife. I wanted to make these changes as easy for her as I could, so the adjustments she was making wouldn't feel too overwhelming. The first few weeks were mainly pan fried chicken breast in olive oil, with either broccoli or asparagus spears on the side.

While I was trying to help her with her new eating habits, I had not changed my own. I would make her a healthy dinner within the timeframe needed to follow the intermittent fasting schedule and then would make myself a pound of fries and a pound of chicken nuggets

NOTES:_____
_____

hours later. In the moment I wasn't thinking about how much more difficult I was making things by cooking foods that would fill the room with the aroma of yummy badness! I did this for about a month before I finally realized how much more difficult I was making this for her. I love my wife, we've been married now for 28 years, and I wanted to be her support, not her undoing and the reason she would return to unhealthy habits.

Once I realized what my actions were actually doing, I decided to join my wife in her journey to improved health. While I am very knowledgeable about health, hydration and nutrition, sometimes it is easier to give advice than take it. I had put on some pounds and was neglecting my own health and I knew if I didn't make a change, the next trip to the E.R. might be for me. I figured if my wife could make this major lifestyle change, then so could I.

She was already showing incredible improvements. She was losing weight, she was increasing her physical activity on an almost daily basis, her mental state was greatly improving and her blood sugar levels were stabilizing. She was doing exactly what she said she was going to do and I was proud of her, while being disappointed in myself for not immediately making the change myself. But better late than never! Her unbridled tenacity and dedicated effort had inspired me and I hopped back on the health train. She inspired the change in me, which inspired this book!

While the rest of the world was losing its mind over the pandemic, we headed down a much different road. Most of my friends were becoming victims of the lockdowns. They were eating poorly, not getting enough sleep and being consumed by the constant barrage of news saying that the world as we knew it was ending.

NOTES:_____

_____

We were self-employed and had been working from home for years, so the lockdowns really didn't faze us like it did most other people. Our personal situation had inspired a focus on health right when we needed it most. Each day we moved forward, while it seemed the rest of the world was taking a step or two backwards. A few other fortunate things had happened for us just before the whole pandemic really started. A few months before the start of 2020 I had purchased an upright freezer so we could take advantage of sales of frozen foods. At the time we had no idea how important that freezer would become!

I was the one who normally did the grocery shopping. Years earlier, when my wife and I first married, money was tight and I started doing coupon shopping in order to stretch our shopping dollar. I took a very business-like approach and became very good at buying a lot of food for very little money. In fact, back in 2002 one of the first books I ever started to write, *Shopping Secrets Revealed*, was inspired by the money I was saving.

Although I never finished that book, the techniques I had learned stuck with me and I continued to be the one who did most of the shopping. As the pandemic continued the shelves of the grocery stores started becoming more and more bare. Luckily, I had the financial resources to buy food in bulk and I just happen to have a freezer to put them in, so I was able to load up on essentials.

During a trip to the store I found ten pound bags of uncooked chicken breast strips for $8.99 per bag. They were tucked away in a part of the store that most people never checked, so as the inventory of the meat department of the store was becoming sparser, I go and literally find hundreds of pounds of chicken at an

NOTES:_____
_____

incredibly low price. Well, I picked up fifteen bags of the chicken. I didn't want to buy it all, as I didn't want to be "that guy", but I also had to watch out for my family, so I bought enough to last us a while. That purchase was a God send! It helped provide what we would need as things got even worse.

Our freezer was stocked and we were eating less, so what we had ended up lasting much longer than in the past, which was exactly what we needed. I think back to so many times during the pandemic that we were so fortunate to be in the right place at the right time. Things were getting better for us. Each day we were making forward progress.

Even my youngest son, who was still living with us, was making excellent progress. He has been singing since he could talk and he was introduced to an online streaming platform called Twitch, which had a karaoke like program called Twitch Sings. His first time using it actually ended up being the same day I took my wife to the E.R. for her eye problem. (www.twitch.tv/thebananiel)

Twitch became exactly the distraction all of us needed. My wife and I could watch our son perform, which we have always loved, and he had a creative outlet when he needed it most. Staying home was tough for him. He was in his twenties, loved to socialize and then the world shut down! The virtual interactions with his new and old friends came at the perfect time and made things much easier for all of us to bear.

I had also reinvigorated my children's book character, the Dream Dragon. As the pandemic was raging on, I knew that children were having a very tough time, so I decided to reintroduce my character, as a way to give

NOTES:_____

_____

hope and direction to kids during this very confusing time.

I started taking the idea of good health even more seriously and invested in some additional exercise equipment, including an elliptical and a treadmill. I started doing a daily workout, usually at the same time my wife was on her exercise bike, and my weight started slowly dropping. I also wanted to be sure to focus on my strength, so I would do between fifty and one hundred incline pushups every day. Kitchen counters, bathroom counters, even the stairs became my workout spot!

If I was going to be serious about regaining my health, I needed to be SERIOUS! Things were going well. We were all feeling better, we were happier and we were staying safe during one of the most confusing times in the history of our world. Then we got the call.

In the evening, roughly four months after his brain aneurysm, my brother-in-law succumbed to the trauma and passed. Getting that call was painful, as we had really hoped he was going to recover. We had spoken to his nurses every day and were encouraged by his progress. Unfortunately, it was just too much for his body and he simply couldn't keep up the fight anymore.

By this time the lockdowns were in full force and no facilities were letting anyone visit their loved ones. He was still in the early stages of recovery and had been moved to a rehabilitation facility in San Diego, CA and we were about an hour north of him. Had it not been for the incredible health changes we had made in the months before, one of us might have ended up hospitalized from the news of his passing. It was hard news, but we somehow kept moving forward.

50

In less than six months I had lost one of my oldest friends, my brother-in-law passed from the brain aneurysm and my wife had a very serious health scare. But somehow we forged forward. We were on the right path and we were staying strong. My family was my rock and without them I'm not sure how or if I would have coped through all of this. But we did not let these things deter us, in fact, they became motivation for us.

We wanted to honor those we lost by becoming the best versions of ourselves. During the same six months my wife went from having A1C's of 10.6 to 5.5. And guess what? She NEVER took one of those Metformin pills! She completely reversed the diabetes by making positive lifestyle changes and much better choices! She lost weight, increased her strength and stamina and feels better than she has in decades! We both discovered our "New You" and we believe you can too!

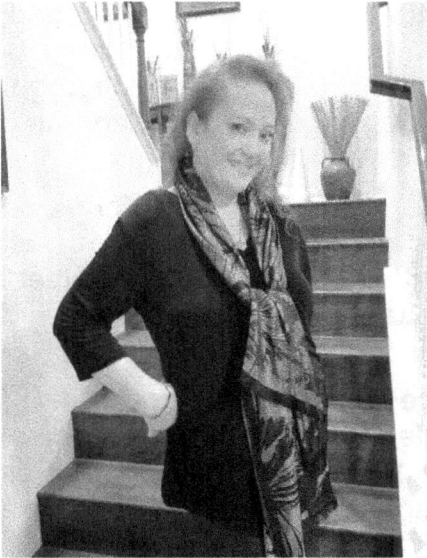

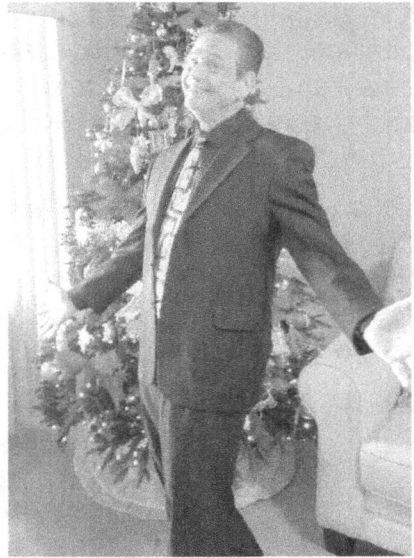

*Life's toughest roads...lead to amazing places!*

51

# THE FEAR OF CHANGE

Okay, I'm just gonna say it, change can be scary. It can make us feel uncertain and out of control. But change is also a natural part of life and can lead to growth and new opportunities. Understanding and managing our fear of change is essential for living a fulfilling life.

One of the main reasons people fear change is because it forces them to leave their comfort zone. We become accustomed to our daily routines and the familiar surroundings that make up our lives. Change disrupts this sense of security and can make us feel uneasy and vulnerable.

Another reason people fear change is because it can lead to the unknown. When faced with a change, we may not know what to expect or how things will turn out. This uncertainty can create feelings of anxiety and fear.

It's also important to note that not all change is bad, change can be positive too. A new job opportunity, a new relationship, or a new home can bring excitement and growth. But even positive change can be scary, as it brings with it new responsibilities and challenges.

To manage our fear of change, it's important to focus on the potential benefits of the change. Remind yourself that change can bring growth and new opportunities. Try to focus on the positive aspects of the change and let go of the negative.

It's also important to practice self-care during times of change. This can include things like exercise, meditation, and talking to a therapist. These activities can help reduce stress and anxiety and provide a sense of stability during a time of change.

NOTES:_____

_____

It's important to remember that change is a natural part of life. Embracing change, rather than resisting it, can lead to a more fulfilling and meaningful life.

## OVERCOMING THE FEAR OF CHANGE

Change is not easy, but most worthwhile things aren't easy, so don't fret. It can be difficult to let go of what we know and embrace something new. But change is also inevitable and necessary for growth. In this chapter, we will explore ways to overcome the fear of change and learn to embrace it as an opportunity for growth and development.

One of the first steps in overcoming the fear of change is to understand that change is a normal part of life. Change can come in many forms, such as a new job, a move, a relationship, or even a change in your personal beliefs or values. It is important to remember that change is not always negative and can bring new opportunities and experiences.

Another important step is to challenge negative thoughts and beliefs about change. Many people fear change because they believe it will lead to failure or disappointment. However, these thoughts are often based on fear and not on reality. It is important to challenge these negative thoughts and replace them with positive and realistic thoughts.

Another way to overcome the fear of change is to take small steps. Change can be overwhelming, so it is important to start small and take one step at a time. This can help you build confidence and momentum as you take on bigger changes.

Practicing mindfulness can also help you overcome the fear of change. Mindfulness is the practice of being

53

NOTES:_____

_____

present and aware in the moment, without judgment. It can help you focus on the present and not get caught up in worrying about the future. Mindfulness can also help you to identify and let go of negative thoughts and emotions that are holding you back from embracing change.

It's important to have a support system in place when facing change. Surround yourself with people who are supportive and encouraging. They can offer guidance and encouragement when you need it most. Overcoming fear can transform you from an acorn of potential to the mighty oak you were meant to be!

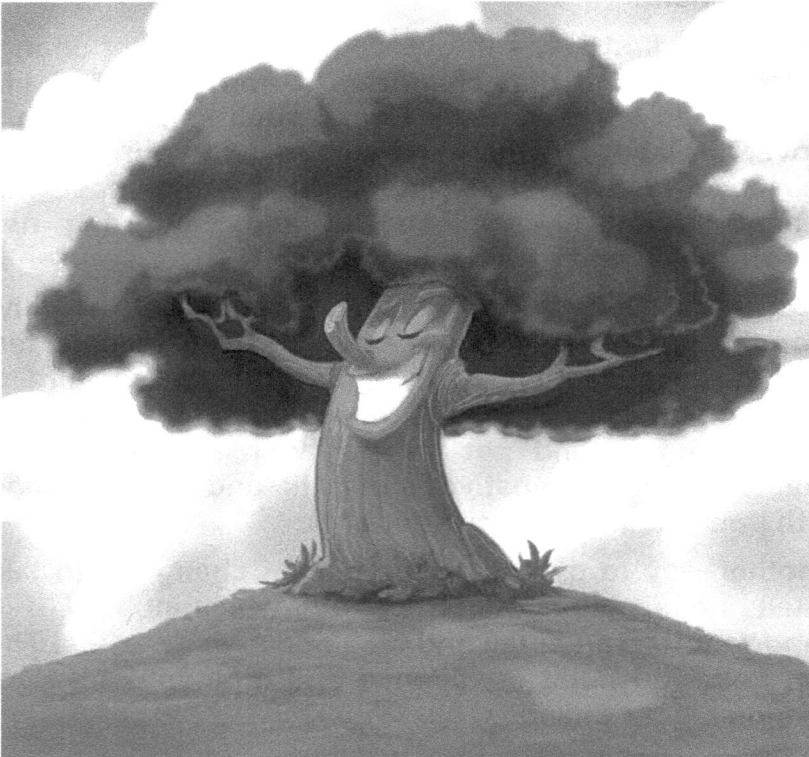

NOTES:_____

_____

# HEALTH THROUGH HYDRATION

Before we jump into this section, I'd like to give a little background about my experience with alkaline ionized water, which will explain why I put so much emphasis on proper hydration when it comes to overall health. I have been a part of the alkaline ionized water industry since 2007 and have earned several million dollars as a result. Being introduced to this water was literally life-changing, so I am compelled to share this information with you, the reader, so you can learn more.

The information in the next five or six pages originally appeared in one of my other books, *Ride The Wave*, which is in its sixth edition and was written for distributors of the water ionizers I represent. I have sold almost 50,000 copies globally, which isn't bad when you consider that the book really only appeals to a very select group of people. *Ride The Wave* has helped tens of thousands of people become healthier and more successful, and I believe that everyone should at least know about this incredible water. Even if you don't decide to try alkaline ionized water, or invest in your own water ionizer, I feel so strongly about the benefits of being properly hydrated that I am dedicating an entire section of this book to this very special water.

Before I continue, I want to explain why hydration has become such a big deal to me. To begin with, water is the most important component to life, at least as we know it. I once said this to a constituent and they replied that they thought air was the most important. This is true, for specific living things, but I was talking about life in general. There are plenty of living things on our planet that do not require air to live, like plant life.

55

So, while air is important to many species, water is an absolute must for every living thing on Earth.

I mean, think about it. When a probe is sent to another planet, like Mars, what do we look for, a soda spring? Or a sports drink river? Of course not, we look for liquid water, because we know how important it is and that liquid water is what we would need to be able to even have a chance at someday colonizing another world. Water is vital for life and good, healthy water is vital for a good, healthy life. I'll get off my soapbox now about the importance of water and will share my journey of discovering a world of water I had never known existed.

Back in 2007 I was introduced to the concept of health through hydration when a close friend and business associate shared information with me about alkaline ionized water called Kangen Water®. I've learned a lot about water and the importance of proper hydration as it pertains to health and will be sharing some of the lessons learned and recommendations about not only how much water a person should consume each day, but the best type of water for optimal results!

When I was introduced to this unique water I had never heard of alkaline ionized water or water ionizers, in fact the only time I had ever heard the word "alkaline" was in regards to batteries. However, I wanted to learn as much as I could, so I rolled up my sleeves and got to work. I immersed myself in everything I could find about water ionizers and the water industry. I started reading as many books as I could find. I also spent countless hours online, digging as deeply as I could, to learn about the history of the technology, the science behind it, the roots of the industry, the claims, the myths, the facts, the benefits, the drawbacks; basically everything.

NOTES:_____

_____

Within a few months I was up to speed and had a pretty well-rounded knowledge and understanding of water ionizers and this special water. I was so impressed with what I had learned and what I had personally experienced that I decided to embark on a business journey with this water. In fact, I ended up becoming a distributor of the water ionizers manufactured by a company called Enagic®. As a distributor I have written two books about the industry and have been a keynote speaker at some of the biggest water ionizer industry events. Now, after nearly two decades, I am taking all my knowledge about hydration and combining it with my knowledge of health, nutrition and finding happiness and putting it in the pages of this book!

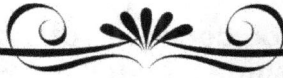

*Life is a mirror.*
*It reflects our choices.*
*Don't like what you see?*
*Make different choices.*
*Change the reflection!*

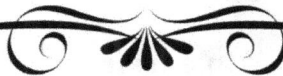

NOTES:_____

_____

# ALKALINE IONIZED WATER - KANGEN WATER®

I try my best to be honest and transparent, so I am going to start this section with some bad news. The bad news is that these water ionizers are incredible devices and the majority of the people who use them love them! You might be scratching your head right now, wondering how that could be considered bad news, so allow me to explain.

You see, while the technology is amazing, unfortunately, just like any consumer product out there, not all water ionizers are created equal. In fact, the vast majority that are available in the U.S. market are inexpensive knockoffs that DO NOT produce the same quality of waters or results as the medical grade water ionizers that I recommend, despite what other manufacturers or sellers claim.

I have almost two decades of experience in this industry, which includes actually testing many of the different brands of water ionizers available today. As such, my opinions on this particular topic are very firmly grounded in facts, not just sales and marketing fluff. That said, the water ionizers manufactured by Enagic®, a Japanese based company who has been in business for over forty years, are the best. If they weren't the best, I would have never connected with them and definitely would not recommend them. But they are the best, so that is my recommendation!

If you decide to invest in a water ionizer to help you stay properly hydrated, then buy one from Enagic®. Don't fall prey to the marketing and sales falsehoods tossed around by other brands and invest in the right machine for you and your family. In fact, if you would like more information, and have not already spoken to or

NOTES:_____

_____

contacted a distributor, I'd be happy to help you. Just send an email to info@powerfulh2o.com to request more information or you can check out my website, www.powerfulh2o.com. If you are already working with a distributor, then please be sure to follow up with THEM. Maintaining the integrity of interest is very important to me, so if you are already working with someone, they should be who you contact!

Before we continue, I want to clarify some things about the name "Kangen Water®". The word "Kangen" does have an actual meaning. In Japanese the word "Kangen" roughly translates to "Return to Origin", this is what the water is trying to help people achieve. This is also a trademarked name belonging to Enagic®. The name "Kangen Water®" refers to alkaline ionized drinking water which is produced by an Enagic® ionizer.

Enagic® understands that the quality of their ionizers sets the water produced apart from that of other ionizers. As such, they decided to actually brand the water produced by their machines with its own name to identify and distinguish it from any other alkaline ionized drinking water. The intention was to establish "Kangen Water®" as the preferred alkaline ionized drinking water; so people can ask for it by name.

Many other companies have successfully used a brand name to identify a specific type of product. When you reach for a Kleenex, you are actually reaching for a tissue made by Kleenex. Have you ever made a Xerox copy on a machine other than a Xerox? One of the most widely recognized is the Band-Aid brand. Their brand has become so well known that most people refer to any adhesive bandage as a "Band-Aid". Following suit with these iconic brands, Enagic® is working diligently to ensure that when people in this market ask for the best

NOTES:_____

_____

alkaline ionized water available, that they ask for it by name, "Kangen Water®"!

Now let's take a look at the different waters these devices produce and how they are most effectively used.

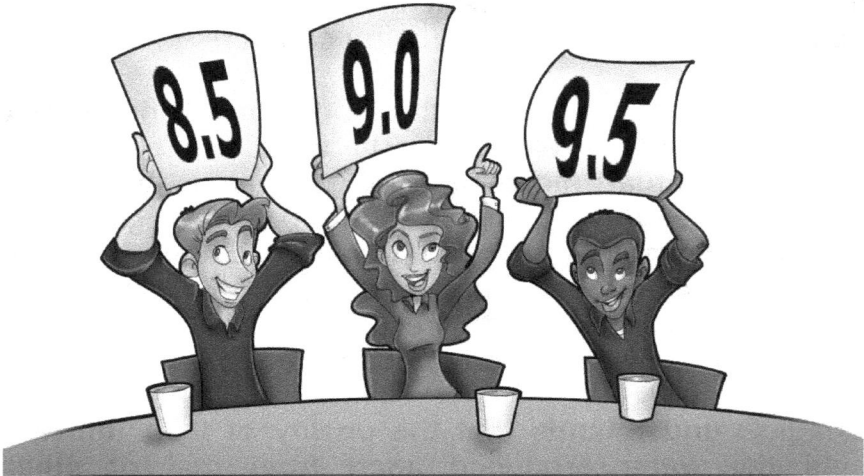

Kangen Water® – There are three grades of alkaline ionized drinking water: 8.5 pH, 9.0 pH and 9.5 pH. These pH values represent alkaline levels that are 50, 100 and 500 times stronger than neutral. How acidic a person is will determine which level of water they should be drinking. Because of lifestyle choices and diet, some people are closer to being balanced, so they may only need the 8.5 pH level; while others are more acidic and need the 9.5 pH Kangen Water®.

Clean Water – This is filtered water that has not gone through the ionization process. This water is mainly used for baby formula, as the body of a baby is already very alkaline, so they really don't need it, until they start eating solid foods.

60

**Beauty Water** – This is water with a pH level of 4.0 – 6.5 and is not intended for drinking. The main use of this water is for topical application to the skin. The pH level is slightly more acidic than the skin, which allows it to tone and tighten. This water is also excellent for certain types of cooking, including boiling pasta and beans.

**Strong Acidic Water** – This is extremely acidic water, with a pH level of 2.6 or less, and is not intended for consumption. With the ability to thoroughly sterilize and sanitize it is perfectly suited for use in any area where contaminants may be found, including kitchens and restrooms. It can also be used to clean foods that may have been exposed to bacteria, including fresh produce and poultry. It is also a very effective hand sanitizer when used to wash hands before food preparation or after handling foods. This water allowed us to never have to worry about running out of hand sanitizer during the pandemic!

**Strong Kangen Water®** – This is extremely alkaline water with a pH level of 11.5 or higher and is not intended for drinking. This restructured water is strong enough to actually emulsify oily spills, but can also be used to clean foods of all kinds, including fresh produce and fish. It is also an excellent all-purpose cleaner, with incredible degreasing abilities. It can also be used to blanch and pre-boil certain vegetables.

The different grades of water produced by an Enagic® water ionizer have many more uses than listed, but these will give you a starting point to understanding the different uses of the water. This is just scratching the surface when it comes to alkaline ionized water, but it's better to start somewhere, than stay nowhere!

NOTES:_____

_____

Now that we've covered the topic of water, I'd like to provide you with some specific recommendations regarding water consumption.

The first, and perhaps most important, is the amount of water a person should drink each day. Contrary to what you may have heard, it is NOT to drink eight glasses of water a day. While this is a good minimum to follow, the reality is that water consumption should be based on the individual, not some standardized, average number. For those who may be stuck on the eight glasses a day, this is one of those common sense moments.

Let's say you have two adults, one is a five foot tall person who weighs 100 pounds and the other is six foot four inches tall and weighs 260 pounds. Now, does anyone really believe that these two people need to consume the same amount of water each day to run the machine that is their body? If you do, I have some swampland in Florida to sell you!

The vast differences in physical size should be more than enough to convince even the most skeptical person to understand that the consumption of liquid water cannot simply be averaged by a number of glasses. So, if the old eight glasses a day is not correct, then what is?

The formula is quite simple and easy to follow once you know it. For best hydration results a person should consume one-half their body weight in ounces of water each day. So a person who weighs two hundred pounds should drink a minimum of one hundred ounces of water each day. Many times when I tell people this they react with shock. They cannot imagine drinking "that much water" in one day. While saying "one hundred

NOTES:_____

_____

ounces" may seem like a lot, once the quantity is put into perspective, it becomes much more drinkable.

Most people in the U.S. are at least familiar with the convenience store 7-11 and that, even if they have never had one, have at least heard of a "Super Big-Gulp", which is a 64-ounce cup, typically filled with a type of soda. That said, most people would agree that they could finish two Super Big-Gulps within 24-hours. Well, if you weigh two hundred pounds and drank two Super Big-Gulps of water within 24-hours, then you would have consumed twenty eight more ounces than the minimum you should consume each day. See, once the amount of water is put into perspective, drinking the correct amount each day becomes much easier to achieve!

So, the next time you step on the scale, remember the number, divide it by two and that is the minimum amount of ounces you should be consuming daily. I say minimum because it is okay to drink more than that. Just be sure to stay hydrated. Since the body is roughly 70% water, with some things, like our blood, being as much as 90% water, it should come as no surprise that proper hydration is vital to health!

I also want to address the difference between beverage consumption and water consumption. Despite the numerous contradicting reports regarding this topic, in my opinion the best way to ensure you are getting enough water to stay properly hydrated is to actually drink the required amount of liquid water you need each and every day. So, if you want a cup of coffee in the morning, fine, just don't count it as part of your daily water intake. The same goes for any other beverage or even watery foods, like certain fruits. I prefer to err on the side of caution, so if I am supposed to drink a

63

specific amount of liquid water each day, then that's what I do and it is also what I recommend. This has worked great for me and should work for you too.

Second is the type of water. I recommend that people at least try alkaline ionized water for their hydration needs, to see what, if anything, it does for them. Even if they do not invest in the technology, I think they should try it. And if you are not going to drink alkaline ionized water, then I recommend just drinking filtered tap water. Based on my research the vast majority of bottled waters are simply repackaged tap water, so why pay a premium for something that is virtually free?

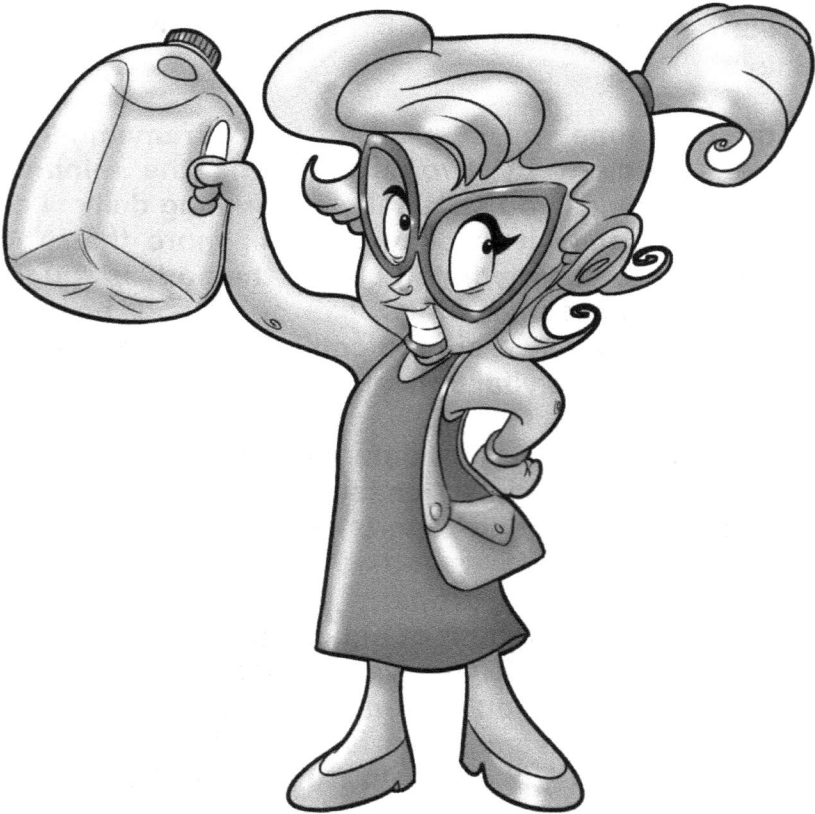

NOTES:_____

_____

# THE STRUGGLE IS REAL!

In the next sections I will discuss some of the challenges faced everyday by consumers, which may be contributing to their health and happiness struggles. These challenges are stemming from the beverage and medical industry, so let's take a look at the two industries I feel are making life much more difficult for just about everyone.

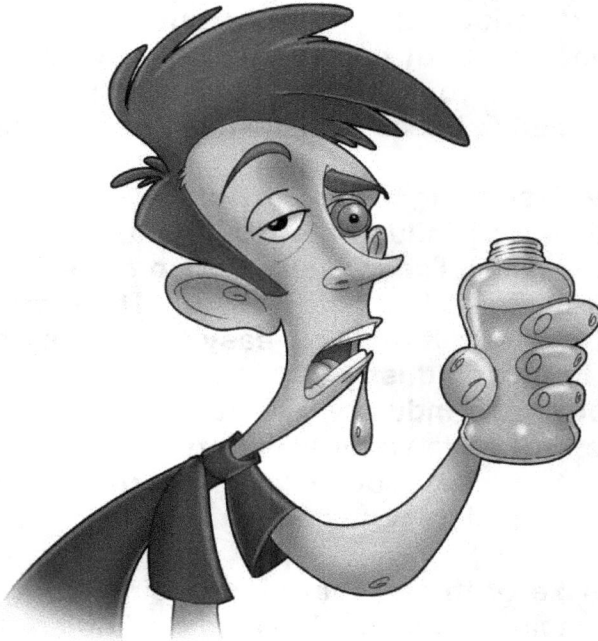

## THE BEVERAGE INDUSTRY – ZOMBIE DRINKS

You are probably wondering why I am dedicating an entire section of this book, about health and self-improvement, to the bottled beverage industry. My journey in the water and health industries have led to realizations about many other things we consume. I've learned about foods and nutrients, but I have also

65

learned negative affects products like soda and other bottled beverages can have on health. Because of this, I felt compelled to discuss the topic, so you, the reader, will be able to make informed decisions when it comes to your health, especially where beverages are concerned.

For many people, grabbing a soda or ordering one at a restaurant has become so engrained that we don't even give how it may be affecting us a first thought, let alone a second thought! Once you have a better understanding about the true nature of these products, you may decide to reduce or eliminate them completely from your eating habits, which I highly recommend!

The very first thing I need to make clear is that the bottled beverage industry is HUGE and there is a lot of money involved. The industry is also more far reaching than just the liquid in a bottle or can. There are so many different facets of it that it is easy to see why the major players in this industry are so powerful. The U.S. bottled beverage industry has been around since 1835, when the first soda water was bottled for sale. But the thing that made soda go mainstream was the introduction of aluminum cans in 1957.

For the sake of this section, I am going to concentrate on two main aspects of the U.S. bottled beverage industry: water & soda. The reason I think it is important to discuss the bottled beverage industry is because they spend an incredible amount of money each year to get consumers to buy their products. They do it through slick marketing campaigns, celebrity endorsements and a variety of other extremely effective methods. Many of these companies have been very successful in creating brand loyalty and some drinks have become a part of many people's daily routines.

66

I try to educate people to some of the hazards of different bottled beverages and these same people can become defensive, because I am challenging what they believe and what they do. This is one of the reasons it is very important to really understand the industry, so you know what you are up against.

The bottled beverage industry spends tens of millions of dollars every year in market research, marketing and advertising. Their ultimate goal is to not only make their beverage a choice of the consumer, but to make it the ONLY choice of the consumer. They strive to create both brand recognition and brand loyalty. A lot of times unhealthy beverages are actually promoted as being good for you, which is why I feel consumers need to know what they are facing, so they can make an educated decision, not an advertised decision!

I believe the complete truth about many bottled drinks will eventually come out and consumers will be more aware of the possible health risks associated with the consumption of these products. But, just like smoking, I think that there will be plenty of people who will disregard the consequences and will continue to pop the top and keep on drinking. In order to fully understand what we are all up against, there are a few important things to know.

First, we know that the vast majority of bottled waters and soda have a pH value that makes them acidic and, most of them have an ORP (oxidation reduction potential) value that makes them an oxidant, which is, of course, bad for the body. Second, we know that there has been a tremendous increase in life style related diseases, especially in children. In fact, according to a prominent child cancer alliance, childhood cancer is

NOTES:_____

_____

statistically the #1 disease related killer of children 15 and under in America.

This is where we have to use a bit of common sense and deductive reasoning in order to make sense of this startling fact. While the statistics are unfortunate, fortunately, the increase has actually happened within a period of time that we can actually see the progression! We can pin point when the increases started, which can then let us figure out what life style changes were happening at the same time and might be related to these changes in health.

The increase in childhood disease has been on the rise for about the past fifty years. Now some will contend that the increase is due to better detection and increased awareness. Unfortunately, this argument is completely unfounded, as the medical community has had all of the necessary testing equipment to discover these conditions for decades. Since we can determine when the increase started, let's consider what changes were happening in America during the same timeframe.

Probably the biggest change was the significant increase in production of and consumption of processed foods and fast foods. Another major change was the introduction of soda as a regularly consumed beverage. For those who are a bit younger, this statement about soda may not make much sense, as we all know that soda in America has been around for well over 50 years. The difference over the past few decades is the way soda ingredients have changed and the way it is now consumed. You see, back in the olden days, soda was considered more of a treat than an everyday beverage. It was something that was available when children had behaved. It was a luxury that was only available every so often, not at every meal.

NOTES:_____

_____

It was the combining of a fast food meal with a soda based beverage that really introduced soda as more of an everyday, every person product , which, again, can be pinpointed to about the mid-1970s as the time when advertising helped this trend sweep across America. In the mid-1980s the trend for bottled waters started to hit, beginning with more affluent people drinking carbonated artisan waters like Pierre in upscale restaurants.

Drinking bottled water started as more of a status symbol than anything else, but it spawned the trend that has now made the bottled water industry one of the biggest industries in America.  If these bottled beverages were not unhealthy, then this would be a trend that would be fine.  However, recent studies have conclude that nearly all of the bottled beverages consumed in the United States pose some sort of possible health issue for the consumer.

With the ingredients in modern day soda it is easy to understand why they might not be very good for us. Heck, some of the listed ingredients read like a chemistry experiment.  Even sodas that claim to be "natural" have preservatives, flavoring, artificial coloring and sugars or artificial sweeteners. Many food and beverage makers use the vagueness that is allowed when using terms like "natural" to market their product.

Unfortunately, the bottled waters out there are not much better.  One of the reasons bottled water ends up being acidic is because of processing requirements.  In order for water to be bottled it is supposed to either be heated to a boiling point, to kill any potentially hazardous contents, or go through a reverse osmosis / distillation process, which will render the water void of any contaminants. Actually, it renders it void of anything!

69

Once the water goes through one of these processes it becomes acidic. Even if minerals are added to the water after processing, which most big bottlers do, the water still remains acidic. Unfortunately, most consumers have no idea that the beverages they know and love may actually be bad for them. I believe, and again this is MY opinion, that within the next decade enough information about the negative effects of some of these bottled beverages will be discovered and that, following suit with the Surgeon General warning on cigarettes, that there will be an actual warning cautioning consumers to the potential harmful effects of consuming the product.

Then, of course, there is the aspect of the environmental impact created by the bottled water industry. Back in the 1950s the bottles were primarily made from glass. Today, the vast majority of the bottled beverage industry uses single use plastic bottles. While these bottles are recyclable, the reality is that only about 27% of plastic bottles are actually recycled. This means that over 70% end up in landfills, highways, waterways and parks, with many ending up in our oceans.

While there is plenty more that we could discuss regarding the bottled water industry, I think that this is enough to give you a foundation of basic information. Obviously, if you want to find out more there are resources everywhere! One of the best is the Internet. If you want to expand your knowledge about the bottled beverage industry, just do some searches on "soda", "bottled water" and "plastic bottles". Just these three key words / phrases could keep you busy for days learning all sorts of things about the industry!

NOTES:_____

_____

# THE MEDICAL INDUSTRY – THRIVE OR ALIVE?

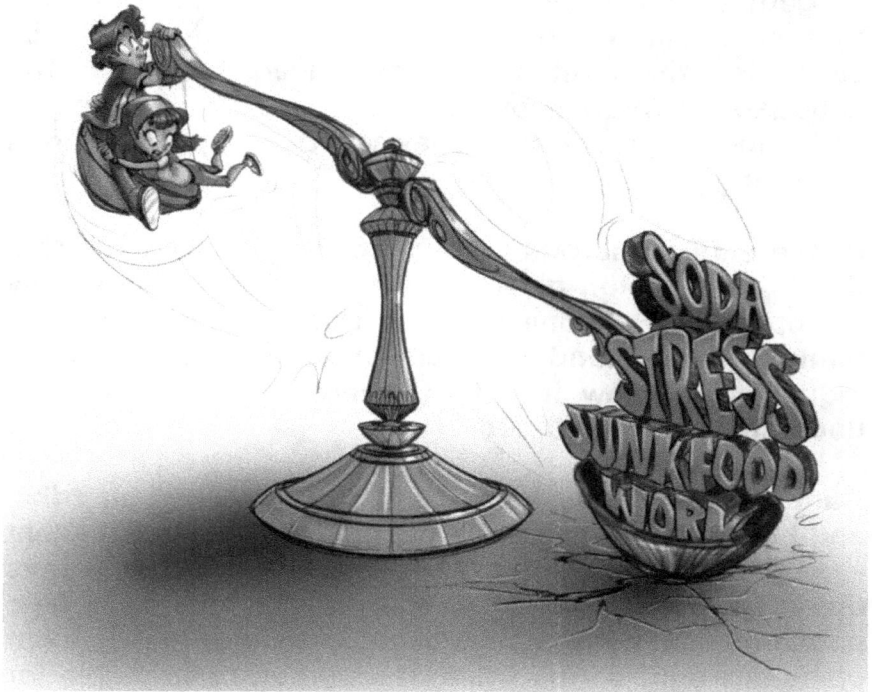

During my nearly two decades in the health and wellness space I have learned many valuable lessons and insight into many aspects of the overall industry. One of these lessons is the harsh reality of the U.S. medical industry. While there is no better place to be if you suffer a medical emergency, in terms of actual "healthcare", the U.S. isn't doing very well. In fact, according to a 2021 report published on WebMD the U.S. health system ranks last out of eleven high-income countries.

The healthcare system in the U.S. has become more sick care than healthcare, which is why it is becoming increasingly more difficult to have faith in the system. It

NOTES:_____
_____

thrives as a result of people being sick, not healthy, so is it really any surprise that people in the U.S. seem to be getting sicker each year? The main portion of the system I am referring to are in what would be considered the traditional "Western Medicine" field. The antiquated approach of diagnose based on symptoms and then prescribe pharmaceutical medications accordingly.

I have said numerous times throughout this book that this is MY opinion on this topic and is not necessarily the opinion of anyone else and this is no exception. I think to understand the current state of the medical industry and how it got to where it is you need to understand how it started.

I am part Choctaw, which is a Native American tribe, and I think the foundations of tribal life are an excellent example of a system that works. You see, in tribal days there were a couple of people in the tribe who held positions of authority and importance. The most obvious would be the Chief, the person responsible for the tribe. But the person who came in a close second to overall importance was the Medicine Man. While it was the duty of the Chief to provide leadership and direction to the tribe, the job of the Medicine Man was to keep the entire tribe healthy.

It is true that being Medicine Man would bring with it a certain level of respect and authority, but I think there is a much more important reason why being a successful Medicine Man would be very important. Was it because of the bigger teepee in the most prime spot of the village? Was it because of the faster, flashier horse he got to ride? Or was it because he actually had a personal, vested interest in the health and wellbeing of every member of the tribe?

72

I believe that the last option makes the most sense. You see, while the members of the tribe were dependent on the Medicine Man to help them stay healthy, the Medicine Man was dependent on the rest of the tribe for his own needs, so if they were in poor health, it would directly affect him. If the Chief were sick, the tribe would be without necessary leadership; if the warriors were ill, the tribe would be without protection; if the hunters were not healthy, the tribe would be without food; if the squaws were sick, there would be no clothes; if the children were sick, there might not be a future for the tribe.

In the tribal world, every one of these things would have impacted the Medicine Man directly, so his overall wellbeing was directly connected to that of the tribe.

Now, let's look at the modern medical industry. Right off the bat, the fact that it is referred to as an "Industry" is a very bad sign. When medicine became an industry, it became a business, which means it centers on profit. I believe that it was the introduction of medical insurance back in the 1950s that really created the current "Medical Industry". It changed the dynamic of medicine being a "calling" into being a "profession".

Believe it or not, there was actually a time when a person would attend medical school because they just really wanted to help people. Nowadays, why do most parents want their kids to become doctors? Because of the PAY!! Not because it is a noble thing to do. It's because it is a way to make good money and lead a more comfortable lifestyle.

Not so long ago, medicine in this country was more like the tribal model than the current model. There was a doctor who would service the needs of people in their

NOTES:_____

_____

own community. You remember, the days of the "house call". Much like the Medicine Man, these community doctors relied on people around them for their own wellbeing. Then communities grew and hospitals were joined by clinics. Then health insurance started limiting which doctors a person could see and patients went from being a familiar face to just another number. The doctor's personal vested interest in the health of each patient had vanished!

Patients have become customers. In business, what are the best kinds of customers? Repeat customers! So, is the medical industry of today really geared towards wanting to keep their customers healthy? Or is it more suited to keeping people just healthy enough to be able to go to work to earn the money needed to cover their co-pay for the office visit?

Ask yourself this question: does it seem like the medical industry wants people to thrive or just be alive?

The answer to this question speaks volumes as to why people in this industry are less than receptive to something that might actually improve the long term health of a person. There is a lot of money in people being, and staying, sick and the reality is that getting and keeping people truly healthy is not financially prudent for the medical industry.

There is another powerful force that greatly influences the medical industry, which are pharmaceutical companies. I know, for a fact, that doctors are encouraged to recommend or prescribe specific brands of medications and that a lot of money is spent by pharmaceutical companies to help ensure that their brand is the one being prescribed.

NOTES:_____

_____

In the paragraph above I said "I know, for a fact", let me explain how I know. A few years back, before I was ever part of the health and wellness industry, my wife worked in the office of a medical doctor's private practice. It was on her very first day on the job that I learned the lengths that pharmaceutical sales reps would go to in order to have their brands be the ones recommended.

When my wife got home from her first day we sat down and she told me all about it. She told me about some of her co-workers, what her basic duties were and, finally, she told me what a great lunch she had and that she did not even have to leave the office to get it.

She went on to explain that a pharmaceutical sales reps had stopped by the office and dropped off lunch for the entire office. I thought that she had lucked out by having her first day coincide with the day lunch was provided for the whole office.

The next day I found out that the lunch had been much more than coincidence. When she arrived home after her second day we chatted again about how things had gone and she, again, ended by telling me that lunch had been provided for the entire office, only this time by a sales representative from a different pharmaceutical company.

By the end of her first week the office had been provided with lunches for the entire staff every single day; each day by a different rep from a different company! And these were not quick, fast-food type lunches. These were full meals from restaurants like California Pizza Kitchen, Pat & Oscars and even P.F. Chang's. It got to the point that she completely stopped making any plans for lunch, as food ended up being provided for the entire office every day that she worked there.

75

I did not realize it at the time, but this ended up giving me some pretty clear insight to just how influential the pharmaceutical companies were becoming when it came to the way doctors were "treating" patients. Just like doctors, prescription drug companies were looking for life long customers, not just temporary users and they would do what they could to jockey into the best position possible.

Now I am sure if any of these representatives were ever asked directly if they ever did anything to try to influence a doctor's decision to recommend their drug, they would say "NO!" or "Of Course Not!". They would probably contend that any recommendation of their brand by a doctor was strictly based on the effectiveness of the medication.

Just so you don't think my viewpoint about this topic is founded solely on biased opinion, please allow me to share with you portions of an article written by Ransdell Pierson and Bill Berkrot, published by Reuters. This article is being referenced strictly for educational purposes.

### *Pfizer paid $35 mln to doctors over 6 months*

*Pfizer Inc on Wednesday said it paid $35 million to some 4,500 doctors and researchers from July through December 2009 for a variety of services, including speaking fees, expert advice and work on clinical trials of its medicines.*

*The world's largest drugmaker last year agreed to pay a record $2.3 billion fine and plead guilty to a criminal charge related to improper promotions of 13 of its medicines, but said the new disclosures were already in the works before that widely publicized settlement...*

NOTES:_____

_____

*...About $15.3 million, or some 44 percent of Pfizer's reported payments over the last six months of 2009, went to about 250 research organizations for clinical trials that began after July 1, or for payments made between July 1 and December 31 for clinical studies.*

*Some 1,500 healthcare professionals were paid an average $5,000 each for expert advice, while 2,800 doctors were paid an average of $3,400 in speaking fees to lecture peers about Pfizer's drugs, the company said. The most highly compensated doctor received about $150,000 during the period, Pfizer said...*

*...Other large drugmakers, including Eli Lilly and Co, have recently begun publishing payments to doctors on their websites. But Neese said its disclosures go beyond those recently established by other companies, in that they include payments for clinical trial research, Neese said.*

*Pfizer said its payment disclosures will become more detailed a year from now, under a corporate integrity agreement with federal health authorities related to the drugmaker's $2.3 billion fine and settlement last summer...*

*...Pfizer in September was slapped with the huge fine by the U.S. government after being deemed a repeat offender in pitching its now-withdrawn Bextra arthritis drug and another dozen medicines to patients and doctors for unapproved uses.*

*Pfizer pleaded guilty in 2004 to an earlier criminal charge of improper sales tactics and its practices have been under U.S. supervision since then.*

*Speaking engagements, in which doctors are paid by drugmakers to discuss their medicines with groups of other physicians, have been among the most controversial industry marketing practices.*

77

NOTES:_____

_____

*By law, companies are forbidden to promote their drugs for uses not cleared by the U.S. Food and Drug Administration. But some companies allegedly have greatly boosted prescriptions for their drugs by allowing or encouraging paid speakers to discuss such "off-label" use of their products...*

So, as I am sharing this information with you what am I really trying to say? What is the point? To me, the bottom line is that medicine is a business and businesses try to make money. The reality is that if your business is to treat sick people, you will not be successful if you make everyone healthy!

If you can wrap your head around this concept, then it may be easier for you to understand why I am not a fan of the medical industry. It boils down to this; the medical industry in the U.S. is great for critical emergency care, but not maintenance of good health. Unfortunately, many people are putting their health in the hands of an industry that does best when their customers are sick.

Remember that personal responsibility section? The fact of the matter is that no doctor, or anyone else for that matter, should be or will be more concerned with your health than you are. You need to assume responsibility for maintaining your health, which means you need to eat right, drink enough of the right water every day, supplement your nutrients if needed, get enough sleep, exercise daily; basically not act like you can do whatever you want without any kind of consequences.

Don't let this industry fool you into believing that they have the answer. Too many people have already followed that prescription and many of those people are paying a painfully heavy price!

78

NOTES:_____

_____

# MENTAL HEALTH

I believe that mental health is a topic most people are still not completely comfortable talking about, mainly because of the perceived negative connotations. Mention the words mental health and suddenly people are thinking about other words like "crazy", "insane", "nuts", etc. But that's not really the mental health I am talking about. I am talking about the aspect of mental health as it pertains to being able to make healthy decisions and actually be happy with who you are.

If you are seeking good health, your mental health is a very important part, in fact it may be the most important part. If your mind, the thing controlling everything about you, isn't healthy, how in the world can you expect the rest of you to be healthy?

It seems everyone these days is trying desperately to be "normal". I think one of the biggest problems with this pursuit is trying to figure out what "normal" actually means. And who exactly is qualified to give that definition or even give advice about mental health? I mean, if we're truly being honest, I don't think there is ANYONE who has everything together and is really in the position to dictate how others deal with mental health. However, I do think that we, as people, have the ability to share strategies or techniques that have made our own mental health journey a little easier, which is what I am going to do.

Will the techniques I have used work for you? Perhaps not, but this is more about gathering ideas and possibilities, than just focusing on a few specific things you can try. Consider this a jumping off point for your own mental health and consider what I've done as suggestions that you may want to try.

NOTES:_____

_____

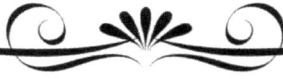

## *Mental Health Helpful Hint*

Making a list each day of what you want to accomplish is a great way to stay on track and on task. Most people are busy and the day can quickly feel like it is getting away from them. Making a list helps keep you focused on what you hope to accomplish, it also allows you to review what you have accomplished each day.

And when you do something that was not on your list, simply add it to the list, so you will remember it was one more thing you accomplished.

If items on your list do not get done, that's okay, simply add them to the list for the next day and do your best to complete them.

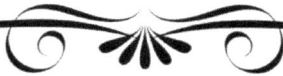

80

NOTES:_____

This section is not going to be very long, as the topic of mental health is not my specific strength; however, I have had enough exposure to psychology and have learned a few things over the years which I feel I can share. These are things that I do which have helped me with my own mental health.

Let's start by reviewing a few of the reasons why mental health is important to overall health. Mental health is an important aspect of overall health and well-being. It plays a crucial role in how we think, feel, and act. When we are mentally healthy, we are better able to cope with the challenges of life, work productively, and make positive contributions to our communities. On the other hand, poor mental health can lead to a range of issues, including poor physical health.

There are several reasons why mental health is closely tied to physical health. First, the brain and the body are closely connected. What happens in the brain can affect the body, and vice versa. For example, chronic stress can lead to physical health issues such as headaches, stomach problems, and a weakened immune system. Similarly, physical health conditions can also have an impact on mental health. Chronic pain, for example, can lead to depression and anxiety.

Another reason why mental health is an important part of physical health is that they often influence each other. Poor mental health can lead to unhealthy behaviors such as substance abuse, overeating, and a lack of physical activity, which can in turn lead to physical health problems. On the other hand, taking care of your physical health through healthy behaviors such as exercise and balanced eating habits can also have a positive impact on mental health.

In addition, mental health problems can be a significant burden on individuals and society as a whole. They can

81

interfere with daily functioning and relationships, and can lead to absenteeism and reduced productivity in the workplace.

Overall, it is clear that mental health is an important part of physical health, overall well-being and, of course, happiness. It is essential to prioritize and take care in order to live a healthy and fulfilling life.

*Excuses make today easy,*

*But make tomorrow harder.*

*Discipline makes today hard,*

*But makes tomorrow easier!*

NOTES:_____

_____

# START WITH YOU

My first suggestion to good mental health is to start with you. What I mean by that is to sit down and have a serious talk with yourself, either literally or figuratively, whichever works best for you. I often talk out loud to myself, as the words resonate with me better when I actually hear them. It's kind of like the old joke about self-employed people talking to themselves.

*"I'm self-employed...*
*I'm not talking to myself, I'm having a staff meeting!"*

So, if you're like me and hearing the words helps you, then talk aloud during this exercise. The conversation you should have may be very difficult for some, but I can assure you that it is extremely important. This is a conversation about accepting yourself. About being able to block out ALL of the negative outside influences that can make us feel like we are not enough or that we have to be someone or something we are not.

I believe that social media, which I feel is named exactly the opposite of what it actually is, has complicated life for millions of people by creating unrealistic expectations of what life is supposed to be. There are way too many pictures of fancy cars and big houses, many of which are not even owned by the people in the pictures!

Many of them are trying to make others think they have some lavish lifestyle, which can make other people feel inadequate and even question their own lives. The irony is that the vast majority of those posting pictures about an incredible life don't actually have an incredible life. In fact, many have a life that is so unfulfilled and empty that they have to try to impress others or show that they

83

NOTES:_____

_____

are "better" than other people with a bunch of "stuff" in order to feel good about themselves. In my opinion many aspects of our world are in a very sad state!

As a society we're becoming so fixated on things like "views" and "likes", as if these things are some sort of indication of the importance of a person. How others, most of which we do not even actually know, respond or don't respond to a comment or post has very little, if anything at all, to do with who you are as a person. Nonetheless, many people are living their lives looking for the approval of perfect strangers, instead of making choices because they are the right ones to make. I guess it is fair to say that digital communication is hindering society.

It's a sad state of affairs, so before you get envious about something or someone you have seen in a social media post, remind yourself that what you're seeing could be nothing but a smokescreen, intended to cover up the dismal, depressing life that the person posting probably has and, in most instances, is not what it appears to be.

So, the first step in dealing with your mental health is to simply be okay with who you are, and I mean the real you! If you don't already, you need to learn how to like yourself, love yourself, respect yourself and realize that who you are is more important than who others think you are! Worry more about your character than your reputation! Reputation is who others think you are; character is who you really are! Strive for character!

Being okay with who I am has taken me quite a number of years, but today I am very happy with the person I see in the mirror. I like the person I am. I know I'm not perfect, but nobody is. Which is why I don't give myself

NOTES:_____

_____

unrealistic goals or expectations, just to end up letting myself down. Why would I do that? I work hard to do my best. I work hard to be better today than I was yesterday and I'll work hard tomorrow to be better than I am today. I help others when I can and I'd like to think I am a pretty decent human being. I feel if I can make minor improvements to myself on a daily basis, eventually I will be the best version of myself. You just have to learn to be okay with who you are while working on who you'll become.

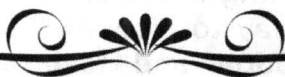

*If you're serious about changing your life,*
*YOU WILL FIND A WAY!*
*If you're not serious about changing your life,*
*YOU WILL FIND AN EXCUSE!*

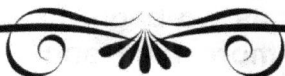

NOTES:_____

_____

# A DIFFERENT KIND OF FASTING: SOCIAL MEDIA

In today's world, social media has become an integral part of our daily lives. From checking our notifications first thing in the morning to scrolling through our feeds before bed, it's hard to imagine a day without it. But what if we took a break from it all? What if we chose to ditch the device and get back to the basics of living? Enter the social media fast.

A social media fast is exactly what it sounds like: a period of time during which an individual abstains from using social media platforms. This can range from a few hours to several weeks, depending on the person's goals and needs.

The reasons for taking a social media fast vary. Some people do it as a way to disconnect from the constant stream of information and take a break from the pressure of always being connected. Others use it as a way to focus on other areas of their lives, such as relationships, work, or hobbies. Still, others may use it as a way to improve their mental and emotional well-being, as the constant social media barrage can be mentally, and even physically, exhausting.

Whatever the reason, a social media fast can be a challenging but rewarding experience. For starters, it can be difficult to break the habit of reaching for our phones and checking social media whenever we have a spare moment. But as we begin to disconnect, we may find that we have more time and energy to focus on other things.

During a social media fast, it's important to set clear boundaries and stick to them. This means not only refraining from using social media apps but also avoiding any other forms of social media, such as watching videos or checking notifications on our

NOTES:_____

_____

computer. It's also important to have a plan for how to fill the time that would normally be spent on social media. This could include reading a book, pursuing a new hobby or rejuvenating an old one, going for a walk, or spending time with friends and family.

As the fast comes to an end, it's important to reflect on the experience. Take note of how you felt during the fast, what you accomplished, and what you learned. And, most importantly, consider how you want to continue using social media in the future. A social media fast can be a powerful tool for understanding our relationship with technology and making meaningful and beneficial changes in our lives.

It is important to note, especially for younger people, that social media is a relatively new addition to humanity. We have no idea what the long-term ramifications to our mental and physical health will be, as it simply hasn't been around long enough to really know. But it is obvious that there are very negative aspects of social media and we should all be cautious.

Humans are social creatures; we need each other in many different ways. To me it is ironic that digital service companies used the term "social media", when most of what happens on these platforms is anything but social. If more aptly named, it would be called "anti-social media", but I guess that wouldn't appeal to very many people.

Be careful not to become so attached to social media that it starts to interfere with your real life. That same life filled with people you love and care about and the friends and family who genuinely care about you!

NOTES:_____

_____

# STRESS – THE SILENT KILLER

Stress is one of the biggest contributors to poor mental health, which is why learning to deal with stress is so important. Stress is a natural response of the body to various challenges and demands, but when it becomes chronic and long-lasting, it can have devastating effects on physical and mental health. In fact, stress is often referred to as the "silent killer" due to its gradual and insidious impact.

The effects of chronic stress can range from mild symptoms, such as headaches and fatigue, to serious health problems like high blood pressure, heart disease, and varying degrees of depression. The body's stress response, known as the "fight or flight" response, was designed to help us survive short-term emergencies. But when stress becomes chronic, the body's stress response remains activated, leading to long-term health consequences.

One of the most damaging effects of chronic stress is on the cardiovascular system. When the body is under stress, the heart rate and blood pressure increase, putting extra strain on the heart and blood vessels. This can lead to an increased risk of heart disease, stroke, and other cardiovascular problems.

Stress can also have a profound effect on mental health. It is a common reason for depression, anxiety, and other mental health conditions. Chronic stress can also interfere with sleep patterns, making it difficult to get the restful sleep necessary for good mental health.

In order to reduce the impact of stress on health, it is important to recognize the signs and symptoms of stress and take steps to manage it. This can include exercise, deep breathing, mindfulness meditation, and seeking support from friends, family, or a mental health

NOTES:_____

_____

professional. Recognizing the signs of stress and taking steps to manage it can help reduce the risk of long-term health consequences. By taking care of ourselves and finding healthy ways to manage stress, we can live a happier, healthier life.

Fortunately, there are many effective strategies for managing and reducing stress. Here are some tips for dealing with stress:

1. Practice relaxation techniques: Relaxation techniques, such as deep breathing, meditation, and yoga, can help reduce the physical and emotional effects of stress. These techniques calm the body and mind and help to release tension and reduce anxiety.

2. Exercise regularly: Regular exercise is one of the best ways to reduce stress and improve overall health. Exercise releases endorphins, the body's natural feel-good chemicals, and can help to reduce tension and anxiety.

3. Get enough sleep: Sleep is crucial for good physical and mental health, and lack of sleep can increase stress levels. Aim for 7-9 hours of sleep per night and establish a consistent sleep routine to help reduce stress.

4. Healthy eating / drinking habits: Balanced and nutritious eating habits can help improve energy levels, reduce stress and support overall health. Try to eat a variety of foods and limit caffeine, sugar, and processed foods. Stay hydrated! The brain is nearly 80% water, so staying properly hydrated is vital for being able to think clearly.

5. Connect with others: Social support is important for reducing stress and improving mental health. Spend time with friends, family, or support

NOTES:_____

_____

groups, or consider seeking the help of a therapist or counselor.

6. Prioritize self-care: Taking time for yourself and doing things that bring you joy can help reduce stress and improve overall well-being. This may include hobbies, reading, or spending time in nature.

These are just a few of the many techniques you can implement to help combat stress. Just remember that if life gets too stressful, step back, take a breath and regroup. Even the worst situations are normally temporary, so stay the course and keep moving forward!

*You are NEVER too old*
*to set a new goal!*
*You are NEVER too old*
*to dream a new dream!*

90

NOTES:_____

_____

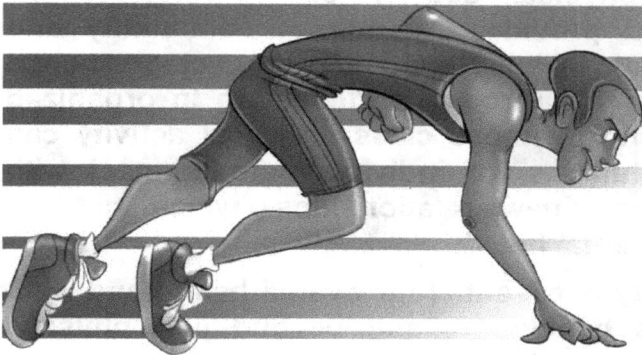

## PHYSICAL ACTIVITY HELPS MENTAL HEALTH

Physical activity is known to have numerous benefits for both physical and mental health. Regular exercise has been shown to reduce the risk of chronic health conditions, such as heart disease, type 2 diabetes, and some types of cancer. In addition to physical benefits, physical activity has been linked to improved mental health and can be an effective tool in managing stress, anxiety, and depression.

Exercise helps the release of endorphins, the body's feel-good chemicals, which can help to improve mood and reduce stress levels. Additionally, physical activity can increase the levels of neurotransmitters such as serotonin, dopamine, and norepinephrine, which play important roles in regulating mood and reducing feelings of anxiety.

Regular physical activity also helps to reduce the symptoms of depression and anxiety by improving sleep patterns, reducing fatigue, and increasing self-esteem and self-confidence. By engaging in physical activity, individuals can shift their focus from negative thoughts and feelings to the sensations and achievements of their bodies, thereby providing a healthy distraction from stress and anxiety.

91

NOTES:_____

_____

Furthermore, physical activity can promote social interaction and provide a sense of community and support, which can have a positive impact on mental health. Whether it's through participating in organized sports or joining a fitness class, physical activity can provide opportunities for individuals to connect with others and form new relationships, which can be beneficial for mental health.

Physical activity is essential for overall health and well-being, and its benefits extend beyond just physical health. Regular exercise can have a profound impact on mental health by reducing stress and anxiety, improving mood and self-esteem, and promoting social interaction and support. Incorporating physical activity into one's daily routine can be a valuable tool for managing and improving mental health.

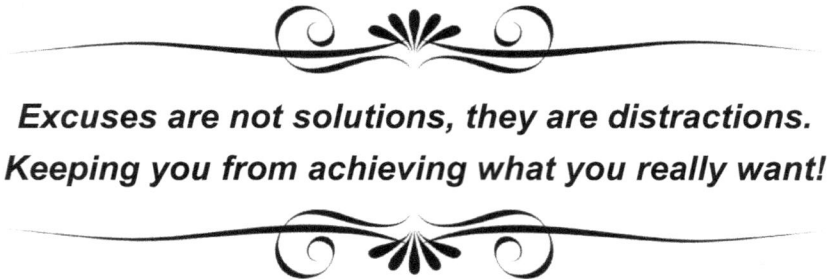

*Excuses are not solutions, they are distractions.*
*Keeping you from achieving what you really want!*

92

NOTES:_____

_____

# EXERCISE AND ACTIVITY

Exercise and physical activity are essential for maintaining good health and well-being. Regular exercise can help prevent chronic diseases, such as obesity, diabetes, heart disease, and certain cancers. It can also improve mental health, boost mood, and reduce stress.

The benefits of exercise are numerous and wide-ranging. For example, regular physical activity can:

- Improve cardiovascular fitness and lung function
- Strengthen muscles and bones
- Improve flexibility and balance
- Boost energy levels and improve sleep
- Help manage weight and prevent obesity
- Reduce the risk of chronic diseases, such as heart disease, type 2 diabetes, and some cancers
- Improve mental health and mood, reducing symptoms of depression and anxiety

In addition to these physical benefits, regular exercise can also have a positive impact on mental well-being. Exercise releases endorphins, also known as "feel-good" chemicals, which can improve mood and reduce stress. Physical activity can also help boost self-esteem and confidence, and provide a fulfilling sense of accomplishment.

Despite the many benefits of exercise, many people still do not get enough physical activity. Inactivity is a major risk factor for chronic diseases and can lead to premature death. To maintain good health, adults should aim for at least 150 minutes of moderate-intensity aerobic activity or 75 minutes of vigorous-intensity aerobic activity per week. To make exercise a

NOTES:_____

_____

part of your daily routine, try to find activities that you enjoy. This will make it more likely that you will stick with it. You can also try working out with a friend or family member, as this can make exercise more fun and provide motivation. Additionally, setting specific, measurable goals can help keep you on track. Below are a few of the many exercise options you can do.

Walking or hiking
Cycling
Swimming
Yoga
Pilates
Resistance band training
Bodyweight exercises (such as push-ups, squats, and lunges)
Dancing
Gardening or yard work
Tennis or other racquet sports
Jogging or running
Jump rope
Aerobics
Calisthenics
Stretching
Weightlifting
Rock Climbing
Roller skating
Ice skating

It's important to note that the best physical activity for you is the one you'll enjoy and do regularly. Everyone is different, so the exercise you choose should be based on your abilities and preference. Consult with a doctor or health professional if you have any health concerns before starting any new physical activity routine.

NOTES:_____

_____

# DIETS

This is not a book pitching some new fad diet, quite the opposite actually. It is an overview of different dietary strategies and explains how anyone can customize their diet to suit their specific needs.

Most fad diets take a one-size-fits-all approach and they usually require a person to adhere to changes that are not realistic for the long term or that are not really all that healthy.

Instead, New You puts a spotlight on some of the most effective dietary choices and explains how you can pick and choose what will work best for you and your body.

## POPULAR DIETS

The following are some of the most popular diets being promoted today. In my own health journey I discovered that while there are lots of different diets out there, despite the countless claims to the contrary, there is no "one-size-fits-all" approach to a healthy diet.

There are several reasons why there is no one-size-fits-all diet that works for everyone.

First, everyone's bodies and nutritional needs are unique. Factors such as age, gender, weight, height, activity level, and overall health all play a role in determining the type and amount of nutrients a person needs. For example, a sedentary adult may have different nutritional needs than an active teenager, and a person with diabetes may need to pay closer attention to their carbohydrate intake than someone without the condition.

Second, individual preferences and cultural backgrounds can also impact a person's dietary habits

95

and preferences. Some people may prefer a vegetarian or vegan diet, while others may follow a specific religion that dictates their food choices. It is important to respect and consider these personal and cultural factors when designing a diet plan.

Finally, the concept of a one-size-fits-all diet ignores the fact that people's bodies and lifestyles can change over time. What works for someone at one point in their life may not be the best fit later on. For example, a person who is trying to gain weight may need to consume more calories than someone who is trying to lose weight. It is important to periodically reassess and adjust a diet plan to ensure that it meets a person's changing needs.

Overall, it is clear that there is no one-size-fits-all diet that works for everyone. It is important to consider individual needs and preferences, as well as the potential for change, when designing a healthy eating plan.

As such, I researched the most popular diets and cherry-picked the parts of each diet which would work best for me and my family. If you are not familiar with the term "cherry-picked", it basically means picking out only the best or most important parts of something and leaving behind the parts that are not needed or do not pertain to your situation.

As you review these different diets / dietary choices, consider what parts may be worth trying and what parts don't really apply to you. You may have to do a bit of trial and error in order to find what works best for you, simply meaning that you may have to implement dietary strategies before you discover if they are actually best for you and your body. Also, be hyper aware of things like fad diets that are not meant for the long-term, as some of these may actually be more harmful than

NOTES:_____

_____

helpful to your health.  Below are the main diets we will be reviewing:

| | |
|---|---|
| Elimination Diet | Sugar-Free Diet |
| Gluten-Free Diet | Crash Diet |
| Ketogenic Diet | Intermittent Fasting |
| Paleo Diet | Fat-Free Diet |
| Blood Type Diet | Dairy Free Diet |

Each of these diets are typically promoted as stand-alone diets, but, based on my experience, the most effective diet is actually a combination of these and maybe even other diets or dietary habits.

Before we review these different diets, let's take a quick look at what the word "diet" actually means.  A diet is the combination of foods that a person consumes on a regular basis. It is the total intake of nutrients, such as carbohydrates, proteins, fats, vitamins, and minerals that an individual consumes to maintain good health. A healthy diet should consist of a balance of different types of foods and provide the body with the nutrients it needs to function properly.

Some people may follow a specific diet for medical or personal reasons, such as to lose weight, lower cholesterol levels, or manage a health condition such as diabetes. Other people may adopt a certain type of diet for cultural or personal preferences, such as a vegetarian or vegan diet. Ultimately, the goal of a healthy diet is to provide the body with the nutrients it needs to maintain good health and prevent chronic diseases.

Many diets have been given a catchy name to try to make them easier to promote and sell, but in my opinion a diet should be more about the individual than a highly

NOTES:_____

_____

specific regiment of food intake suggested by someone else. If your name is Jack, you should be on the "Jack Diet", meaning that you should be eating a combination of foods that provides the best outcome for Jack. If your name is Jill, then it would be the "Jill Diet", and so on. There is so much information about food available that there is no reason for a person not to customize their eating habits to what will be absolutely best for them.

Don't get caught in the "diet" trap, customize your eating habits to fit your needs, as there is only ONE you!

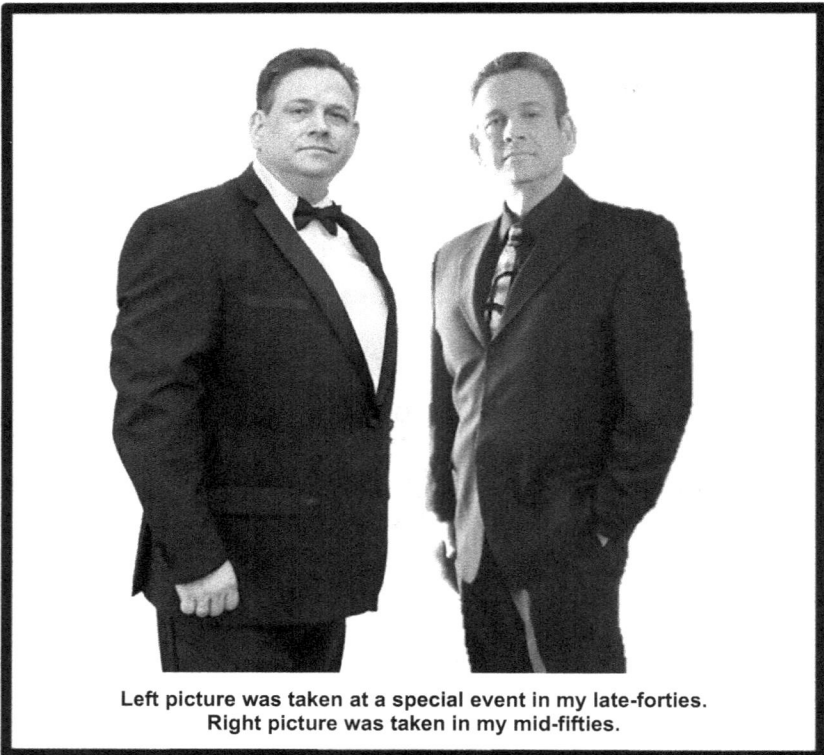

Left picture was taken at a special event in my late-forties.
Right picture was taken in my mid-fifties.

98

Diet has truly become a four letter word, heck the word "die" is literally the root of the word, so how good can a "diet" really be? Instead, I'd like to suggest that you change your mindset by using a different word choice and refer to your eating habits as just that...eating habits.

In order for change to last, you must develop new habits, not simply change things for a short time and then think you can return to your old, bad habits, it doesn't work like that. So NO MORE diets, which are temporary! Let's commit to long lasting, customized healthy eating habits that you can actually stick to, because this is how you'll discover the New You!!

Just so there is no confusion, I will be referring to many of the popular "diets" using the word diet. I don't want anyone to be confused by me saying to stop using the word diet and then calling all of these diets. This is how they are known, so that's why I will call them that. My suggestion is that you stop referring to what you are eating as your "diet" and, instead, use the phrase "eating habits". The word "diet" just has too many negative connotations.

## Elimination Diet

An elimination diet is a dietary plan that involves temporarily removing certain foods or food groups from a person's diet in order to identify any potential food sensitivities or allergies. The goal of an elimination diet is to identify the specific foods that may be causing unwanted symptoms or reactions, such as digestive issues, skin problems, or other health concerns.

To follow an elimination diet, a person typically removes the most common allergens or potentially problematic

NOTES:_____

_____

foods from their diet for a set period of time, usually between two to six weeks. After this period, the person slowly reintroduces these foods one at a time, while monitoring their symptoms to determine which foods may be causing problems.

An elimination diet is often used as a diagnostic tool in cases where a person has unexplained symptoms or suspected food intolerance, but it can also be used as a way to improve overall health and well-being. This can be a very effective way to identify foods that you should consider cutting out of your eating habits.

This is exactly what I did, which is how I discovered that I have a gluten sensitivity. I completely cut out wheat based products from my eating habits and within a few weeks I noticed marked improvements. When I consumed wheat products after that I noticed headaches and joint pain. While everyone may have a different reaction or no reaction at all, I discovered mine simply by temporarily eliminating gluten. Once I identified my sensitivity, I simply removed those foods from my eating habits permanently.

## Gluten-Free Diet

Being gluten-free may be a challenging and sometimes isolating experience, especially if you are new to the gluten-free lifestyle or if you live in a community where there is limited awareness or understanding of gluten sensitivity or celiac disease. However, with some education, planning, and patience, it is possible to lead a healthy and satisfying gluten-free life. I experienced this myself when first staring with gluten-free eating habits, but I adjusted to it quickly and it became not only an important part of my overall eating habits, but very easy to follow.

100

NOTES:_____

_____

## What is Gluten?

Gluten is a protein found in wheat, barley, and rye. It is responsible for the elasticity and chewiness of bread and other baked goods, as well as for the thickening and binding properties of sauces, soups, and other processed foods. For people with celiac disease, an autoimmune disorder, ingesting gluten can damage the small intestine and prevent the absorption of nutrients from food. For those with non-celiac gluten sensitivity, gluten can cause a range of digestive and non-digestive symptoms, such as bloating, abdominal pain, diarrhea, constipation, fatigue, and even headaches and joint pain.

## Going Gluten-Free

If you have been advised by a healthcare professional to follow a gluten-free diet, it is important to understand that this means eliminating all sources of gluten from your diet. This includes not only obvious sources like bread, pasta, and baked goods, but also less obvious sources like sauces, soups, processed meats, and even medications and supplements that may contain gluten as a filler or binding agent.

It can be overwhelming to try to identify and eliminate all sources of gluten from your diet, especially if you are used to eating a lot of processed foods or if you eat out frequently. Here are some tips to help you get started:

- Educate yourself about the sources of gluten. There are many online resources, books, and support groups that can provide information about gluten-free living, including lists of gluten-free foods and brands.

- Learn to read labels. All packaged foods in the US are required to list the major allergens, including wheat, on the label. However, not all products will be labeled as "gluten-free," so it is important to

101

familiarize yourself with the various terms that may indicate the presence of gluten, such as "wheat," "barley," "rye," and "malt."

- **Focus on whole, unprocessed foods.** Many whole, unprocessed foods are naturally gluten-free, such as fresh fruits and vegetables, meats, poultry, fish, and eggs. These foods can form the basis of a healthy, gluten-free diet.

- **Experiment with alternative grains.** There are many grains and grain-like seeds that are naturally gluten-free, including quinoa, rice, corn, oats (if labeled as gluten-free), amaranth, millet, and teff. These grains can be used in place of wheat, barley, and rye in a variety of dishes.

- **Eat out with caution.** Eating out can be challenging on a gluten-free diet, as cross-contamination is a common concern. It is best to stick to simple, plain dishes, such as grilled meat or fish with vegetables, and to communicate your dietary needs to the server and chef. Some restaurants may have gluten-free menus or options available, but it is always important to confirm that they are prepared in a safe and separate environment.

Managing a gluten-free eating habit takes some effort and planning, but with time and practice, it can become second nature. Remember, just like all aspects of your health, if you are unsure of how changes to your eating habits may affect you, consult with a healthcare professional or registered dietitian for personalized advice and support.

NOTES:_____

# Ketogenic Diet

The ketogenic diet, also known as the "keto diet," is a high-fat, low-carbohydrate diet that has gained popularity in recent years as a weight loss and health improvement strategy. The goal of the keto diet is to get the body into a state of ketosis, in which it burns fat for fuel instead of carbohydrates.

To follow the keto diet, you need to significantly reduce your intake of carbohydrates and increase your intake of fats. This usually involves eating fewer than 50 grams of carbohydrates per day, which is a very low amount compared to the 250-300 grams of carbohydrates that the average person consumes. In contrast, the keto diet emphasizes the consumption of healthy fats, such as those found in avocados, olive oil, nuts, and seeds.

One of the benefits of the keto diet is that it can lead to rapid weight loss, as the body burns fat for energy instead of carbohydrates. It may also improve certain health markers, such as blood sugar and cholesterol levels. However, it's important to note that the keto diet may not be suitable for everyone, and it should be followed under the guidance of a healthcare professional.

There are a few potential downsides to the keto diet. One concern is that it can be difficult to stick to, as it requires a significant change in eating habits and may not provide enough variety in terms of nutrients. Additionally, the diet may not be suitable for athletes or people with high physical activity levels, as the body may not have enough carbohydrates to fuel intense exercise.

Overall, the keto diet may be a useful tool for some people looking to lose weight and improve their health, but it's important to consult with a healthcare

NOTES:_____

_____

professional before starting any new diet. It's also important to remember that, as with any diet, the key to long-term success is finding a sustainable and healthy eating plan that works for you.

## Paleo Diet

The paleo diet is a dietary approach that involves eating whole, unprocessed foods that are similar to those that were consumed by humans during the Paleolithic era. This diet emphasizes foods such as meats, seafood, vegetables, and fruits, and limits the consumption of grains, legumes, and processed foods. The paleo diet is typically low in carbohydrates, as it excludes many carbohydrate-rich foods, such as grains and legumes.

Low carbohydrate diets can be effective for weight loss and improving markers of health, such as blood sugar and cholesterol levels. However, it is important to note that these diets may not be suitable for everyone and may be associated with certain risks and side effects, such as nutrient deficiencies and an increased risk of heart disease. It is important to speak with a healthcare provider before starting a low carbohydrate diet and to ensure that all nutrient needs are being met.

## Blood Type Diet

The blood type diet is a dietary regimen that proposes that people's blood type determines what foods are most suitable for them to eat. The idea behind the blood type diet is that people who follow a diet that is tailored to their specific blood type will experience improved health and wellness.

Proponents of the blood type diet argue that many different blood types are based on location and have evolved to process certain types of foods more efficiently, and that following a diet that is suited to a

NOTES:_____

person's blood type can help them achieve optimal health. They claim that individuals with different blood types have different metabolic and digestive characteristics, and that these differences can be exploited through diet to improve health.

There are four main blood types: A, B, AB, and O. According to the blood type diet, people with type A blood should follow a vegetarian diet that is high in grains and legumes and low in meat and dairy products. People with type B blood are advised to follow a diet that is high in meat and low in grains, legumes, and dairy products. People with type AB blood are advised to follow a diet that is a mixture of the type A and type B diets, while people with type O blood are advised to follow a diet that is high in protein and low in grains and dairy products.

The blood type diet is another that I have personally incorporated into my eating habits. After reviewing what foods were advised, neutral and those I should avoid, I simply removed the ones I should avoid. This included pork and wheat products. I will mention that I did not remove all of the foods I was advised to avoid, but I believe removing the ones I did has helped me.

## Sugar-Free Diet

The term "sugar free" is used to describe food and drinks that do not contain any added sugars. This includes white sugar, brown sugar, honey, and other sweeteners that are added to food and drinks to make them taste sweeter. Sugar-free products may still contain naturally occurring sugars, such as those found in fruit, milk, and some vegetables, but they do not contain any added sugars.

Sugar-free products are often marketed as a healthier option for people looking to reduce their sugar intake.

NOTES:_____

_____

Some people choose to consume sugar-free products because they are trying to manage their blood sugar levels, such as those with diabetes or pre-diabetes. Others may choose sugar-free products for weight management purposes, as excess sugar intake can contribute to weight gain.

It's important to note that just because a product is labeled as sugar free does not necessarily mean that it is a healthy choice. Many sugar-free products are still high in calories and may contain other ingredients that are not healthful, such as artificial sweeteners or other additives. It is always a good idea to read the nutrition label and ingredient list on any food or drink product to understand exactly what it contains.

Crash Diet

A crash diet is a type of diet that involves making rapid and drastic reductions in calorie intake in an attempt to lose weight quickly. Crash diets are often characterized by extremely low calorie intake, and may involve cutting out entire food groups or eating a very limited range of foods. These diets are often marketed as quick and easy ways to lose weight, but they can be dangerous and unhealthy, as they do not provide the necessary nutrients that the body needs to function properly. Crash diets can also cause rapid weight loss, which can be unhealthy and may not be sustainable in the long term. It is generally recommended to avoid crash diets and instead adopt a healthy and balanced diet that provides the body with the nutrients it needs while also promoting weight loss.

Crash diets are diets that promise rapid weight loss in a short period of time, usually through drastic reductions in calorie intake or the elimination of certain food groups. These diets are often not sustainable in the long

NOTES:_____

_____

term and can be harmful to your health. Some examples of popular crash diets include:

1. The Atkins Diet: This diet involves cutting out carbohydrates and increasing your intake of protein and fat.

2. The Dukan Diet: This diet involves four phases, including an initial phase where you only eat lean protein.

3. The Grape Diet: This diet involves cutting out all grains and starchy vegetables, and only eating vegetables, fruits, and protein.

4. The Lemonade Diet: Also known as the Master Cleanse, this diet involves drinking a mixture of lemon juice, water, cayenne pepper, and maple syrup for several days.

5. The Military Diet: This diet involves a strict 3-day meal plan that includes specific foods in specific quantities.

It's important to note that crash diets are not recommended for long-term weight loss or overall health. It's always best to talk to a healthcare professional before starting any new diet or exercise program.

<u>Intermittent Fasting</u>

Intermittent fasting is a pattern of eating that involves alternating periods of eating and not eating, also known as fasting. It is a popular approach to health and wellness that has gained popularity in recent years due to its potential benefits for weight loss, metabolic health, and overall well-being.

There are several different approaches to intermittent fasting, including the 16/8 method, in which individuals

NOTES:_____

_____

fast for 16 hours and eat during an 8-hour window; the 5:2 diet, in which individuals eat normally for 5 days and restrict their caloric intake to 500-600 calories for 2 non-consecutive days; and the one meal a day (OMAD) approach, in which individuals eat only one meal per day.

One of the primary mechanisms by which intermittent fasting may benefit the body is through its effects on metabolism. During periods of fasting, the body is forced to use stored energy sources, such as fat, for fuel. This can lead to weight loss and improvements in body composition. Intermittent fasting may also increase insulin sensitivity, which can help regulate blood sugar levels and reduce the risk of type 2 diabetes.

In addition to its potential effects on metabolism and weight management, intermittent fasting has also been shown to have other potential health benefits. Some research suggests that it may improve markers of heart health, such as blood pressure and cholesterol levels, and may also have anti-inflammatory effects. It may also have a positive impact on brain function, including improving memory and cognitive performance.

However, it is important to note that more research is needed to fully understand the effects of intermittent fasting on the human body. As with any change in diet or exercise routine, it is always a good idea to consult with a healthcare professional before starting an intermittent fasting program.

Additionally, intermittent fasting may not be suitable for everyone. Certain individuals, such as pregnant women, children, and people with certain medical conditions may want to avoid fasting or consult with a healthcare professional before starting.

NOTES:_____

_____

I implemented intermittent fasting into my dietary lifestyle choices and it has been very effective. I have lost weight and kept it off. My first meal of the day is at 2:00 PM and my last meal is typically between 6:00 PM – 7:00 PM, but I really try not to eat after 7:00 PM. If I am having a "hungry night", what I refer to as a "hunger hurdle", I will make some lightly salted popcorn, which always curbs my appetite.

If you decide to do the same I would recommend that you keep control of what you are eating by making the popcorn "old style" on the stove top, using cooking oil and popcorn kernels you picked out. I do NOT recommend using microwave popcorn, as there are typically lots of additives, salts and even sugars in certain brands. Making popcorn from scratch allows you to keep control, including the amount of salt you add.

## Fat-Free Diet

Fat-free refers to a product that contains no fat or has had the fat removed. This can be achieved through various methods such as using low-fat or fat-free ingredients, removing visible fat from the product, or using processing techniques to remove fat. Fat-free products are often perceived as being healthier or having fewer calories than their full-fat counterparts, but this is not always the case. It is important to read nutrition labels and ingredient lists carefully to understand the nutritional content of a product.

Low-fat refers to foods or diets that are lower in fat content compared to similar foods or diets. Fat is a type of nutrient that provides energy and helps the body absorb certain vitamins. However, consuming too much fat, especially saturated and trans fats, can increase the

NOTES:_____

_____

risk of certain health problems, such as heart disease and obesity. Therefore, it is often recommended to choose foods that are low in fat as part of a healthy diet. Low-fat foods usually contain 3 grams or less of fat per serving.

## Dairy Free Diet

Dairy-free refers to food and beverages that do not contain any milk or milk-based ingredients. This includes milk, cheese, butter, yogurt, and cream. People who follow a dairy-free diet avoid these products for various reasons, such as allergies or sensitivities to lactose (a sugar found in milk), ethical concerns, or health and wellness goals. There are many alternatives to dairy products available, such as plant-based milk made from nuts, seeds, or grains, and dairy-free cheese and other products made with non-dairy ingredients. It's important to note that being dairy-free does not necessarily mean a product is vegan, as it may contain animal-derived ingredients such as eggs or honey.

There are many reasons why people choose to follow a dairy-free diet. Here are the top five reasons:

1. Lactose intolerance: Lactose intolerance is the most common reason people choose to follow a dairy-free diet. Lactose intolerance occurs when the body is unable to digest lactose, a sugar found in milk and other dairy products. Symptoms of lactose intolerance include bloating, gas, diarrhea, and abdominal pain.

2. Allergies: Some people are allergic to proteins found in milk, such as casein and whey. These allergies can cause symptoms like hives, rash, swelling, and difficulty breathing.

110

3. Ethical concerns: Some people choose to follow a dairy-free diet for ethical reasons, such as a concern for animal welfare or environmental sustainability.

4. Health benefits: Some people believe that a dairy-free diet can have health benefits, such as aiding in weight loss or reducing the risk of certain diseases like acne, cancer, and osteoporosis. However, it is important to note that a well-planned dairy-free diet can still provide the necessary nutrients for good health.

Some people may have difficulty digesting lactose, the sugar found in milk and other dairy products. This can cause symptoms like bloating, gas, and diarrhea. Some people may also be allergic to the proteins found in dairy products, which can cause a range of symptoms including hives, coughing, and difficulty breathing.

There is also some evidence to suggest that high intake of dairy products, particularly high-fat dairy products, may be associated with an increased risk of certain health problems. For example, some studies have found that high intake of dairy products may be linked to an increased risk of prostate cancer and ovarian cancer. Other research has suggested that high intake of dairy products may be associated with an increased risk of acne.

It's important to note that the relationship between dairy and health is complex and there is ongoing research in this area. Some people may be able to include dairy products in their diet without any problems, while others may need to limit or avoid dairy due to intolerance or allergies. It's always a good idea to talk to a healthcare provider or a registered dietitian if you have concerns about your diet or if you're considering making any changes to the way you eat.

NOTES:_____

_____

I was originally convinced that adhering to a dairy-free diet was beneficial to health as a result of meeting one of the premier gastroenterologists in the world, Dr. Hiromi Shinya. Dr. Shinya based his dietary philosophy on a unique perspective of his experience in examining over 300,000 patients during his lengthy medical career. Dr. Shinya was the medical pioneer of endoscopic removal of pre-cancerous polyps from the colon. This technique, referred to as "The Shinya Method", revolutionized medicine making it far safer than the previously used invasive major abdominal surgery.

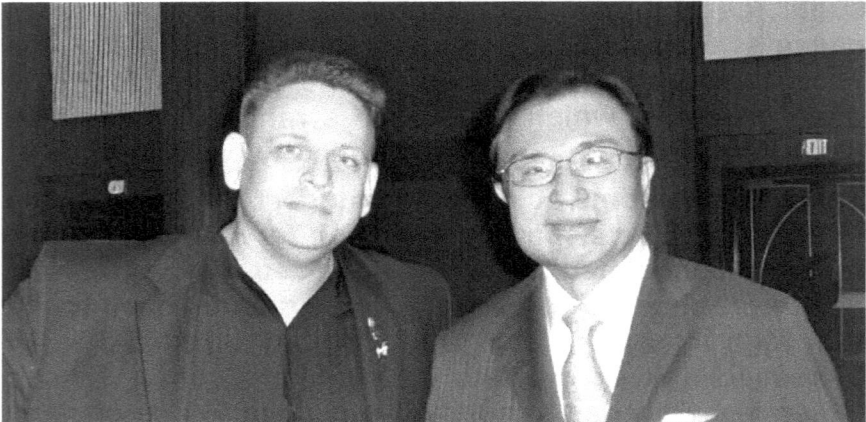

Gerald Kostecka and Dr. Shinya at an alkaline ionized water convention where both were keynote speakers

Although Dr. Shinya has made major contributions to surgical treatment, his true passion was the relationship between diet and intestinal health. It led him to the discovery of the important role that both food and digestive enzymes play in overall digestive health.

What does Dr. Shinya say regarding a dairy-free diet? Let's look at the information Dr. Shinya provides in his book, *The Enzyme Factor*.

112

*"Milk and other dairy products are often difficult to digest and create gut issues for many people. This is especially prevalent in individuals who are Asian or Black given the higher probability to be lactase deficient in the intestinal lining."*

I know that Dr. Shinya was one of the most knowledgeable people in the world when it comes to digestion, so it was easy for me to listen to his advice! When something makes sense and is also corroborated by the top expert in the field, I don't need much more than that to give it a try.

As a result, I am mostly dairy-free, with the exception of the occasional dairy based cheese every now and then. We all have our "exceptions". Based on my own experience and research, and the recommendations of Dr. Shinya, I typically recommend that a person try to be dairy-free as much as possible.

My main reasons are:

1. A person is not a baby cow, which is the animal cow's milk is intended for.
2. Cow's milk is only consumed by the animal it is intended for roughly a year, not for the rest of their life.
3. Cow's milk is meant for an animal with four stomachs.
4. Baby cows drink cow's milk in order to gain substantial amounts of weight in a short period of time, typically between 300 – 500 pounds in less than one year.

Based on these, and many other reasons, I do not drink dairy and try to limit my dairy intake to only every now and then. I recommend that people adhere to a dairy-free diet as much as possible.

113

Combining the most effective "ingredients" of different diets to create your customized eating habits can become a recipe for success!

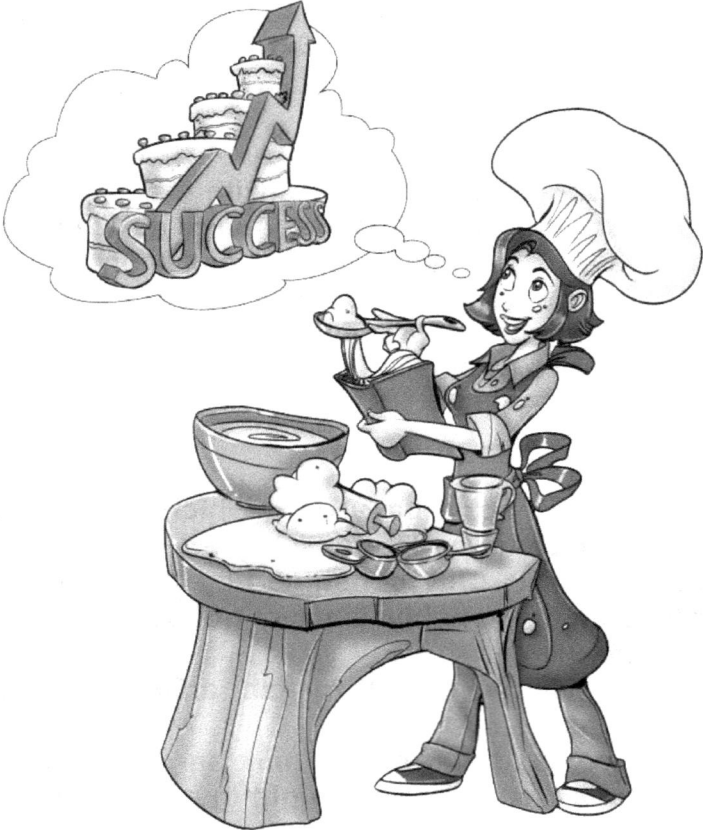

NOTES:_____

_____

# FALLING BACK INTO BAD HABITS

Let's be completely honest, if you're reading this book, you have probably developed some habits that are not really the best for your health and happiness. We've all done it, including me, so you don't have to beat yourself up about it. But do recognize that it will be very easy to fall right back into those bad habits, especially when you first start on your journey of making positive lifestyle changes. It's important to put those habits as far behind you as possible. The further you get from them, the less likely you will be to return to them.

Most people go through a "honeymoon" period with just about anything new in life. This is usually right at the beginning of starting something new; when they are 100% committed, completely dedicated to doing what they need to make a positive change in their life. This period can last a few days, weeks, months or even years, but, unfortunately, most people will eventually start slipping back into their old, bad habits again. This is why it is so important to stay focused on your goals and stay true to what you want. Until a person has developed a new lifestyle choice into a habit, meaning that we do what we should without even thinking about it, even the best of us is susceptible to falling back into our old habits.

This does not happen because we want it to, it happens because change can be hard and humans basically do things based on one of two reasons: something brings us pleasure, so we pursue it; or something causes pain, so we avoid it. This is really why creating a new habit is so difficult. Change usually involves some level of "pain". It may not be physical pain, it may be mental. Just the thought of making a change is uncomfortable for some people, and discomfort is a form of pain! But if you want this to work, you must be willing to endure the

115

_____

pain of change, so you can experience the new pleasures that positive change has the potential to bring.

According to a study published in the European Journal of Social Psychology, it takes 18 to 254 days for a person to form a new habit. The study also concluded that, on average, it takes 66 days for a new behavior to become automatic. This means that you will probably need to give yourself at least two months for these changes to take hold, so make sure your honeymoon period lasts at least two months!

The hardest thing about personal change is that no one is forcing you to do it, which is why it is so easy to fall back into bad habits. You have to learn to become accountable to yourself and not accept your own excuses. The harsh reality is that no one will be more concerned with your health than you are; nor should they be. Your health, or lack thereof, is ultimately your responsibility and until that fact is accepted and embraced, improved health will most likely not stick.

YOU have to decide to be healthy!

YOU have to create positive habits!

YOU have to commit to the process!

YOU have to want a healthy lifestyle!

This is exactly the reason that this book is titled NEW YOU, because that is what we are trying to accomplish. Let's be 100% honest, if the old you was working, you probably would never have picked up this book in the first place, so this is your reality check. You have to want what positive change can bring you more than you want the things which contributed to your current health situation. It's not easy, but it's worth it!

This section is not meant to lecture, but to serve as a warning. This process is not easy, but nothing in life

NOTES:_____

_____

that is worthwhile is!  So be warned, while this book is meant to help you find the NEW YOU, the only person who can screw this up, is also YOU!

You must not become complacent!  Most people will tell themselves, "I would never...", but if we're being honest, not only will we, but we already have numerous times, and we'll do it again if we're not paying attention!

My hope is that this section ends up being irrelevant and a moot point.  Just be aware of the very real possibility of slipping4 back into bad habits and how important it is to correct your course as soon as you discover it is happening.  Having a lapse of judgement, a moment of weakness or simply falling back into an old habit will happen, I know for a fact!  The important thing is how you deal with it, that you address it immediately, take back control and get then get yourself back on track.

People seem to be more mindful and worried about keeping their phone charged, than keeping their health charged.  I know that we live in a digital age, but that doesn't mean that all things digital are the most important thing in the world.  Heck, your phone won't really matter that much if you are too sick / ill to use it!

We all need to get our priorities straight!!

NOTES:_____

_____

# THE DREADED SCALE

Anyone who has ever had an issue with weight will tell you just how much they hate the dreaded scale. It is often seen as the bearer of bad news, instead of the helpful tool that it should be. That's correct; I called it a tool, even when most consider it some evil thing put on this planet to torment them.

Most people who decide to try to lose weight will suddenly become connected to the scale, even though they probably seldom ever stepped on a scale before making the decision to lose weight. Unfortunately, this can actually become counterproductive when it comes to a weight loss journey. This is because every day weigh-ins can make it seem like you are making very little progress, because not much happens on a day-to-day basis, so it can look like you're not making progress, which can lead to giving up. Remember that change comes with time, so you have to be patient, which includes using a scale.

People with a weight issue did not create that issue overnight. It usually takes years and years for weight to be gained and health to decline, yet people think that losing that same weight that it took so long to gain will happen quickly. It won't, so ground your expectations in reality instead of desirability. This is not to say you won't be able to lose noticeable amounts of weight once you start on a NEW YOU journey, but it will probably take time, so be ready.

As I mentioned earlier, a scale is a tool and like any tool it works best when you use it correctly. Here are a few tips to help you use this important tool, without wanting to throw it out the window!!

NOTES:_____

_____

### Tip # 1 – Know a few things about weight and the body.

Most people do not know that a gallon of water weighs eight pounds. Why is this important? Well, let's say that you have a nice big glass or a few glasses of water before weighing yourself; think your weight will be accurate? Of course not! The scale does not know the difference between your body weight and the added weight of the water you just drank, so it will reflect your weight, plus the weight of the water you just drank, which could easily be a few pounds, giving an inaccurate reading of YOUR actual weight.

### Tip # 2 – Weigh yourself weekly.

Instead of jumping on the scale every day, and setting yourself up for possible failure, designate a day of the week to be your scale day. This should be the only day you use the scale. A weekly review will give you a much better feel for your progress versus daily checkups that sometimes don't reflect your effort. If you are the same or gaining weight, then simply turn up your efforts a bit more and keep working. The scale is simply to let you know where you are in your journey. If what you see is not where you want to be, then make the necessary adjustments to get back on track.

### Tip # 3 – Review weight in the morning.

If you want to get the most accurate reading of your weight, then weigh yourself in the morning. Exactly when you weigh yourself will be based on your schedule, but the best time to weigh yourself will be before you eat or drink anything and, if possible, after you have had your morning bowel movement. This will give you the most accurate measurement of your weight, as what you will be weighing is mostly YOU, not you and stuff in you that won't be later.

NOTES:_____

_____

Tip # 4 – Weigh yourself nude.

Clothes have weight, so if you step on the scale wearing anything but your birthday suit, the number you see will include the weight of your clothes. Since we're trying to get the most accurate reading of what you weight, not you and your outfit, we need to drop the clothing and hop on the scale "all natural"!

These simple tips will help turn that dreaded scale into the bringer of good tidings and the tool that it was always meant to be!

## UNDERSTANDING YOUR RELATIONSHIP WITH FOOD

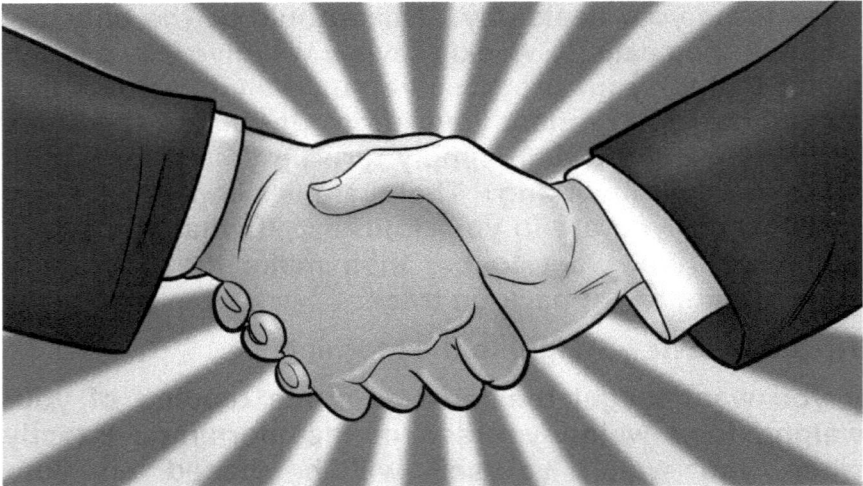

Your relationship with food is just like any other relationship! It can be healthy and good for you, or it can be toxic and bad for you, it really depends on how YOU approach and deal with the relationship. If you want to take control of your health, you MUST be willing to not only ask the tough questions of your relationship, but you MUST be willing to accept the answers, no matter how difficult they may be!

120

I'm not a psychologist, but I know that if a person is having a toxic relationship of any kind, a change needs to be made. When it comes to what you eat, this type of change usually starts by understanding your part in an unhealthy relationship with food. If you discover that your relationship with food is leaning towards the toxic side, which it does for most people who pick up this book, then you'll need to identify the toxic parts of your eating habits and decide to make a change! It might be hard, but you may just need to "break-up" with the foods that are toxic for you!

## DINING OUT

If you are like a lot of people, eating out at restaurants or having food from a restaurant delivered is probably something you do more than you should. According to a Zagat study, average Americans dine out or order delivery five times a week; numbers are even higher in cities like New York and Los Angeles. While they might be tasty, most restaurant food is not the highest quality, as they do need to make a profit on each meal, so most of what you eat will have a quality level just good enough to justify the price you're paying. They are also usually very high in sodium and other preservatives, to limit spoilage and reduce cost. Basically not all that good or healthy for you!

While the food at most restaurants may result in poor health, if eaten in excess, the reasons for wanting to eat out may be much more deeply seeded than most people would expect. This is when the dysfunction of a relationship with food may start to appear.

It is very possible that a person who feels a lack of control in their life will go out to eat simply as a way to feel a sense of control. This is not to say that this is the

NOTES:_____
_____

case for every person, every time. I am also not saying that this is a conscious thought or decision, as many of the things we do are done without us even realizing there is a reason for it, this is more of an example of a "why" when it comes to the habits of some people. Identifying the reasons behind your habits is the first step to understand what needs to be done to make a positive change.

If you, like most everyone these days, have a dysfunctional relationship with food, it is important to fix that relationship if you ever want to find your best you. If a person is using food as a "drug", understand that it can be just as dangerous as any drug that is being misused. People "overdose" on food all the time. It just doesn't usually result in immediate issues. The opposite is actually true, which is why it is so much more dangerous.

The negative effects of a dysfunctional relationship with food typically takes years to manifest, making identifying the issue that much more difficult. If we went from healthy to unhealthy overnight, we'd probably address the issue much sooner. It can take years to notice the negative changes, which allows us to continuously get used to our current condition. You didn't gain those extra pounds overnight, which means it will take time to lose it, but once you realize there is an issue, it is vital for you to take action! Healthy eating starts with you controlling your food, NOT your food controlling you!

NOTES:_____
_____

# WHAT YOUR FOOD SHOULD BE

I think it is safe to say that food has become an important part of life and I mean beyond the needs of the body. There are entire television networks dedicated to food. It's no wonder that people have such a tough time with food, as we are constantly bombarded with food related information and are tempted with delicious foods almost anywhere we go. For the sake of this book and making positive changes, let's get back to basics when it comes to food.

First and foremost, food is fuel. It is the fuel for the body and for the mind. Just like fuel for your vehicle, we need to put the correct amounts and type in our engine for it to perform at peak levels. It's funny how many people give more thought and attention to the fuel they put in their car than the fuel they put in their body!

You are the most important "machine" in your life. Not your phone, not your television, not your computer, not your car...YOU! That said, I urge you, the reader, to give yourself the attention you deserve, by making you as important as something like your car! I'm pretty sure you wouldn't put honey in place of motor oil and lemonade in place of gasoline, as it would destroy your automobile. Yet we will fuel up with fast food, preservatives and refined sugars with little to no thought of the damage being done to our body. The true difference is that if your vehicle breaks down, you can always get a new one. When the body breaks down, well, typically that is the end of the line!

Hippocrates (Hip-pock-crow-teas), who is often referred to as the Father of Modern Medicine, famously said, "Let thy food be thy medicine and let thy medicine be thy food." Let's discuss some of the specific things you should be looking to get out of the food you consume.

123

NOTES:_____

_____

## Nutritious

The majority of what you eat and drink should be beneficial to the body. Like fuel for your car, what you put into your body will directly affect how your body runs and operates. This is an important reason that the foods you eat should have sufficient nutritional value to promote the health of your body. Unfortunately, many foods these days are almost completely void of any nutrients and are loaded with empty calories, refined sugars and preservatives. Part of getting healthy is getting educated. You may need to become proficient with reading food labels and understanding food in order to ensure you are getting what you need nutritionally.

## Tasty

Food should have a pleasing taste, as it makes eating it that much easier and more enjoyable. This is one of the key reasons many "healthy" foods are frowned upon; they don't taste very good. Well, times they are a changing and many of the not so tasty healthy foods have been improved to make the taste more pleasant and inviting. For the past twenty years the idea of health has increased, which is why many of these foods have been revamped. They taste better so people will want to eat them.

Unfortunately, some of these same changes have turned what once was healthy food into foods that sound healthy but are not actually healthy. Processed Vegan foods are an excellent example. Contrary to popular belief, something being Vegan does not make it inherently healthy; it just means it does not contain animal or animal by-products. I have seen plenty of processed Vegan foods at the grocery store that are loaded with sugars, so be sure to not assume

NOTES:_____
_____

something is a healthy choice simply because of a dietary type or catchy product name.

Also be cautious to stay away from processed foods high in refined sugars, High Fructose Corn Syrup and sodium; another reason to become skilled at reading food labels. Many of the foods which contain these particular ingredients have been made to seduce your taste buds, but they are typically not good for health. So, if you have to indulge in these tasty and tempting, yet not at all good for you foods, do so in moderation and infrequently. You must keep control of the food you eat...DO NOT let it control you!

<u>Social</u>

Many times eating is a social activity. In fact, I think that most people would agree that sitting down to a good meal with friends or family is just about the best way to enjoy a meal. Unfortunately, many people use a social eating occasion as an excuse to forget all about their healthy eating habits. It may be because it can be more difficult to stick to a specific eating habit when going to a restaurant or a party or wherever the social occasion may take you or perhaps we get swept up in the spirit of the occasion and forget about what is best for us.

I am often amused when people say things like "...I was just treating myself..." when they talk about eating something that they know they shouldn't. Keep in mind that most of the time these "treats" are things that are pleasing to the taste and which also are only actually enjoyed for a few seconds, maybe a few minutes. But then the treat is over and the reality sets in. Just be sure that if you decide to treat yourself, that you really think about what harm that treat might be doing. And realize that the enjoyment of the treat is fleeting, while the negative consequences may be long lasting. I mean are you really doing yourself any favors by eating

NOTES:_____

_____

something that is absolutely delicious, but that ends up messing up all the hard work you've been doing? Don't allow yourself to undermine your efforts any more than you would allow someone else to mess up your hard work. You deserve better, even from yourself!

When in social settings you have to be sure to remind yourself that a gathering is not an excuse to throw caution to the wind. Show the same kind of restraint and self-control that you would if you were eating at home. Your location has nothing to do with making the right choices. Even if every person around you is indulging in foods, eating like there is no tomorrow, this is not an invitation for you to do the same. It may take a bit more self-control, but you can do it!

So, before grabbing that additional item or something that you know is not good for you, take a moment and really think about it and try your best to do what is best for you, not what sounds good in the moment. Impulsive actions rarely have fantastic outcomes! The benefits of those moments are fleeting, while the negative effects can last for years. This can take a high level of self-control, but once you develop these actions into habits, it is much easier to achieve.

Just remember that humans are basically motivated by two types of actions; the pursuit of pleasure or the avoidance of pain. For the most part, every action we take will have a foundation on one of these two primal desires. You just have to be wise enough to be able to see both sides of the coin when faced with a decision that seemingly offers both, pleasure and pain. While that sweet, tasty dessert may bring you some pleasure, probably a few seconds worth, it will most likely create much more in the way of pain, but in the moment all we seem to be able to recognize is the pleasure aspect.

NOTES:_____

_____

Decisions should be based on complete information, so if you're going to eat that dessert, at least acknowledge the aspect of the pain it might cause you and then really weigh the consequences of that decision. You know yourself better than anyone else, so you should know the things that motivate you, to do both healthy and unhealthy things. Don't make it any easier on yourself to make unhealthy choices than you have to. In fact, you should make the unhealthy choices so difficult that it is easier to simply make the healthy choice!

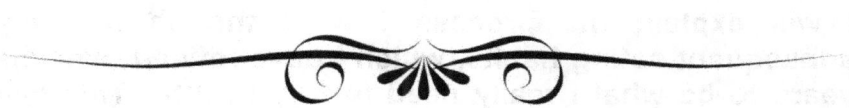

---

**Being healthy is a personal choice**

**You can either do what's good for you**

**Or you can do what's bad for you**

**You'll either enjoy the outcome**

**Or suffer from the results**

**The choice is yours**

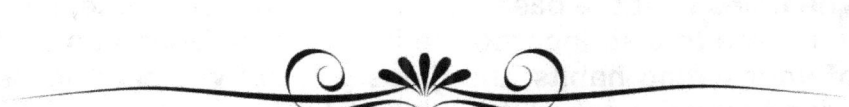

---

NOTES:_____

_____

# FIGURING OUT NEW EATING HABITS

Now that you've reviewed different dietary plans, it's time to customize your approach and figure out your new eating habits. This process takes time, as you may need to experiment a bit, which may require you to remove foods from your eating habits and then reintroduce them, to see how they affect you. This may be the only way you will know what is working for you and what is actually working against you.

I will explain the process I went though and my subsequent eating habits, which I have refined over the years to be what I really need for my health. This can serve as an example of what has worked for me. Please remember that this process and the end result will be different for everyone, even people who live together and eat the same things. We are all different, so even though our habits may seem identical to someone else, it does not mean that the way those habits are affecting us are the same. They can be very different!

Here is a breakdown of my current eating habits. I share this as an example of what I ended up implementing after a lot of trial and error. This IS NOT intended to provide a template for anyone else to duplicate, as what works best for me will not work for everyone. Remember, we are customizing our eating habits to maximize results for each individual, not a one-size-fits-all approach.

Meal Times: As I have mentioned before, I have incorporated intermittent fasting into my eating habits. The times I eat are based on my personal schedule, so if you were to also incorporate intermittent fasting as part of your eating habits, the times you eat will need to be based on your schedule. I am not a "morning person", meaning that I do not wake up early in the morning. I

NOTES:_____

_____

typically wake up between 9:00 AM – 10:00 AM, so this is where my day starts. If you wake up earlier or later than this, you will need to adjust your times to make sense for your schedule.

My fasting schedule is based on a 19 – 20 hour fast, with meal times starting at 2:00 PM and usually ending no later than 7:00 PM, with the occasional lightly salted, stove top made popcorn, for those hard to deal with hunger hurdle nights. This is an advanced fast that takes time to adjust to. Most people are fine with a 16:8 fast, meaning they do not eat for 16 hours and only have meals during a specific 8 hour window.

I usually start my day with a big glass of fresh alkaline ionized water. Drinking water first thing in the morning has numerous benefits for the body and mind. Firstly, drinking water on an empty stomach helps to rehydrate the body after a long night of sleep. This can boost energy levels and increase overall alertness. Additionally, drinking water in the morning can help to flush out toxins and improve the function of the digestive system. It can also stimulate the metabolism, leading to increased weight loss and improved digestion.

Moreover, drinking water first thing in the morning can also improve skin complexion by hydrating the skin from within and reducing the appearance of wrinkles and fine lines. Furthermore, drinking water in the morning can also boost the immune system, reducing the risk of illness and helping the body to fight off infections. Overall, drinking water first thing in the morning is a simple and effective way to improve health and wellness.

I usually follow my morning glass of alkaline ionized water with one or two cups of black coffee, but I try hard to not exceed that amount. Drinking coffee has both

NOTES:_____

_____

pros and cons. On the positive side, coffee is a great source of caffeine, which can increase energy levels, alertness, and physical performance. It also contains essential vitamins and minerals, such as vitamins B2, B3, and B5, manganese, and potassium. Studies have also suggested that coffee consumption may lower the risk of certain diseases. Additionally, coffee has been shown to improve mood and reduce symptoms of depression.

On the other hand, too much coffee can lead to jitters, anxiety, and insomnia, as well as increased heart rate and blood pressure. It can also cause acid reflux and digestive problems. Furthermore, caffeine in coffee can be addictive and reducing or stopping coffee consumption can result in withdrawal symptoms. So, if you're going to drink coffee, do it in moderation.

If you add any of the numerous flavorings, syrups or creamers that are available to your coffee, pay attention to what is in whatever you may be adding. Many people do not realize that what they are adding to their coffee may have as much sugar as a cupcake, so don't fool yourself into thinking you're making healthy choices by ignoring the reality of what you are adding to your morning cup of coffee. Pretending that what is essentially a milkshake is actually a cup of coffee is not doing anyone any good at all!

After my water and coffee, I start my work day. I have found that staying busy is a great way to curb my desire to eat. I think this may be why so many people had such a hard time during the lockdowns of the pandemic. People who are usually at their place of employment were suddenly working from home, where the easy availability of the refrigerator created a massive temptation to snack, sometimes throughout the entire day. Self-control can be hard, especially if there is no one around. A lot of times social pressures inspire us

NOTES:_____

to not do things when around other people, like not eat something every fifteen minutes!  But when the only person around is you, it is much easier to simply do what you feel in the moment.  Times like these are when self-control is the most crucial!

I usually have my first meal at 2:00 PM.  I say "usually" because just like anything in life, there are exceptions. If I have something going on that makes it necessary to eat a little earlier or even a little later, that's okay.  It's about being as consistent with your schedule as possible.  My first meal generally looks like a normal lunch, although sometimes I will be in the mood for some good, old fashioned breakfast foods.  Like a veggie omelet, some turkey bacon, a few pieces of gluten-free toast and some fresh fruit.  When not in the mood for breakfast for lunch, I usually have a turkey wrap on an almond flour tortilla, some plantain chips, a small amount of mixed nuts and an apple or some other fresh fruit.

I used to have a veracious appetite.  I could consume a lot of food at one sitting.  But as I started reducing the quantity of food I ate and started losing weight, smaller amounts of food would satisfy my hunger.  This is a natural part of the process.  But it is important to make sure that you are maintaining the proper amount of nutrients each day.  If you reduce the amount of food you are eating, make sure you offset the reduced nutrients with some sort of supplement.

The idea is to be healthy, not just skinny.  During my journey I got down to 174 pounds, which, for me, was too much weight loss.  I started feeling fatigued and even lethargic.   I realized my body needed more nutrients, so I made additional adjustments to maintain my healthy weight range, which is between 190 – 200 pounds.  This range will differ for every person and you are the best gauge of your healthy weight range.  You

131

will discover that there is a weight range that makes you feel the best. Staying within that range will help you be healthier and happier, because you will feel better.

My meal window is usually only around four to five hours, so I don't typically need to eat between meals. However, sometimes I am feeling hungry, so I will grab a piece of fruit or some other healthy food to tide me over until my dinner. Snacking is fine, as long as the snack makes sense. Eating a bag of potato chips between meals does not make sense, so be realistic and mindful about what you eat between meals.

My dinner, and last official meal of the day, is usually eaten between 6:00 PM and 7:00 PM. While there are some circumstances which can push this back a bit later, I find it important to keep my final meal within this timeframe.

I want to address something that will most likely come up if you decide to try intermittent fasting. The first few days, or even weeks, will be difficult. So much so that you may be ready to throw in the towel and raid the refrigerator. To this all I can say is, be strong. I know the temptation and the desire to relieve your discomfort will be overwhelming. It will not be easy. But being easy has never meant it is the best thing to do. In fact, I think most people would agree that the best things in their lives came as a result of hard work, effort and determination. This is just one more of those times. The discomfort will pass and you will be okay. I know from my own personal experience that the feeling of accomplishment will far outweigh the discomfort.

I also want to mention that if you do falter, it's not good, but it's okay. Moments of weakness do happen. It's how you respond to them that is important. If you have a moment of weakness, recognize it, accept it and move forward. The most important thing is to not let a

NOTES:_____

_____

moment of weakness become an excuse to stop trying. Don't let those moments take control. You're in control, so if you suffer a setback, just regroup and take back control. You have that power.

Just to be clear, I went through this exact issue, which is why I know it can and most likely will happen. When I first started intermittent fasting I struggled, a lot! I would actually wait until my wife went to bed and would then stealthily eat something else. It was like I was trying to trick myself into believing I was following my fast, because my wife thought I was. Actually, it was one of these occasions that was my breaking point.

My wife had gone to bed and I was up watching some late night shows, when a slight feeling of hunger appeared, one of those hunger hurdles. Almost out of pure habit I went to the refrigerator and started looking for something to eat. Undecided, I grabbed a package of lunch meat and started eating a few slices while I was deciding what I was actually going to eat. After eating what felt like one or two slices of the lunch meat, I looked down and realized I had eaten almost half the package. As I looked at the half eaten package of lunch meat in my hand a feeling of utter disappointment surged through me. This became one of those pivotal life moments for me.

"What the frick is wrong with you, Jerry? You're stronger than this! Your wife has been kicking butt with this and you're down here sneaking around like a thief in the night. Are you fricking kidding me? She deserves better than this and so do you! Put that down, close the fridge and pull your head out of your butt!"

And with that, I stopped the late night cheat eating. But I didn't say "frick" or "butt", my language with myself was a bit harsher, I think you can probably figure it out. I've mentioned before that I talk out loud to myself all

NOTES:_____

_____

the time, as hearing the words help them solidify in my mind. This was simply an unfortunate conversation I needed to have with myself!

It was my own wakeup call that, while my wife would be disappointed with me, I needed to hear because the person I was really letting down was me. You can't fool yourself forever! I will not accept being treated with such disregard and disrespect, especially from myself. I deserve better and demand it. Holding yourself accountable for your actions is truly the only way you can make forward progress, so don't let yourself off the hook, but you don't have to beat yourself up either!

Unfortunately, many people let one moment of weakness destroy all the work they have done. They allow their setback to fill their mind with thoughts of self-doubt and unworthiness. Convincing them that they are not strong enough and that they should just give up.

That would be like thinking that if you're ever late for work, you should quit your job. Would that make any sense? Of course not! So why would a moment of weakness be an indication of your worth? It's just a temporary setback; as long as that's all you allow it to be. So be realistic and understand we, as people, are not perfect, we all will make mistakes, we all will make poor decisions and we all will experience setbacks. These do not define who you are or what you deserve, so just give yourself a break!

What's funny is I ended up telling my wife about my weakness inspired pivotal moment and her response made me remember exactly why I married her and why I love her so much. "I knew. Did you really think I didn't notice how much food was gone from the time I went to bed until I woke up the next day?" When I asked her why she didn't say anything, her reply brought me to

NOTES:_____

tears. "I believe in you and knew you would get yourself on track. I'm glad I was right." I apologized for lying to her and thanked her for allowing me to figure this out myself. Sometimes we have to fall a little to remind ourselves how high we've climbed! That said let's get back to the final meal of the day.

My dinner is usually a protein, chicken or beef, along with a healthy portion of vegetables and sometimes a starch, like potatoes. No matter what you eat, the most important thing is that it is sensible. If you are feeling a little more hungry than usual, make a dinner salad to accompany your meal. If you are feeling sluggish, maybe have a vegetarian night to help flush your system. Your body will tell you what it likes and what it doesn't, if you listen! Please note I said your body, not your mind!

Your mind may tell you that all it wants are the things that are the worst for you, and if that happens, DO NOT listen! If you pay attention your body will send signals letting you know what works and what doesn't. When you find things that work, stick with them. When you find things that don't work, eliminate them from your eating habits, it's that simple.

One very helpful kitchen appliance I have added to my regular routine is an air fryer. It has allowed me to greatly reduce the amount of fried foods I eat, while still allowing me to enjoy the feeling that my food has been fried. If you don't have an air fryer, based on my personal experience, I would recommend getting one. I guess this is a good time to also mention that I do not use a microwave oven.

My family stopped using a microwave oven many years ago and I'm glad we did. I discovered that using a microwave oven can present potential health hazards. Prolonged exposure to microwave radiation can lead to

NOTES:_____

_____

eye damage and an increased risk of cancer. Microwaving food in plastic containers can result in the leaching of harmful chemicals such as BPA and phthalates into the food. Additionally, the heating process can result in a loss of some of the food's nutrients, particularly heat-sensitive vitamins like Vitamin B12 and Vitamin C. Besides the convenience of heating something quickly, I really haven't missed not using a microwave oven at all.

There are occasions that I am hungry a few hours after my final meal. Health and happiness are about balance, so I understand I can't just ignore this feeling. I cover this in greater detail in an upcoming section called Eating Habit Exceptions, but I will touch on this briefly now.

When I find myself wanting more food after my dinner I will make some lightly salted, cooked on the stove top popcorn. I do have a cut off time that I won't even do this, which is 10:00 PM. If it's past 10:00 PM, I can wait until the next day to eat something. I'll just have a glass of alkaline ionized water, which helps satisfy that "empty" feeling in my stomach.

Now let's take a quick look at the different diets that I used to customize my actual eating habits. There are actually quite a few! I'll start with the things I eliminated from my eating habits.

I stopped eating pork and eat very little dairy, except for the occasional cheese, which I address in the next section. I do not drink any soda, sports drinks or energy drinks. In fact, I mainly drink alkaline ionized water or beverages I can make with my water. In fact, even when I dine out, I bring my water and simply ask for an empty glass when asked what I'd like to drink. I've been a water drinker since I was a kid, so this is actually very easy for me. Every now and then I will

NOTES:_____
_____

indulge in an organic 100% pure orange or grapefruit juice, but not much more than that.

I've incorporated aspects of the blood type diet, which are foods that are either recommended, neutral and those I should avoid, based on my blood type. I discovered I have sensitivity to wheat gluten, so I also eat gluten-free. I use parts of the keto diet and low-sugar diet. I have a couple of other diets peppered in there as well, including eating primarily organic, but these are the main ones I have used to create my customized eating habits. I have found that while no single dietary plan has worked for me, the combination of numerous dietary strategies has worked great!

I can actually stick to this because it's not a diet, it's my eating habits. I have enough variety to keep me satisfied and have incorporated the parts of many different diets that work best for me. It's been great!

## EATING HABIT EXCEPTIONS

It is said that there is an exception for every rule and, since you are making the rules for your new eating habits, then you can also make the exceptions! While I wouldn't create a lot of exceptions, it is nice to create a few, right as you get started, so when the time comes for you to break your own rules you know what to do and don't end up going too far backwards.

I will share with you a few exceptions I have in my eating habits, but these will vary from person to person. The main idea is to have a few exceptions you can fall back on, but limit the amount of exceptions you have and really try to stick with your new eating habits.

My first exception is in regards to dairy. While I have cut a solid 97% of dairy from my eating habits, I do have

NOTES:_____

_____

the occasional cheese. I've tried plant based cheeses and they simply do not satisfy the craving when I am in the mood for cheese, so when I feel like I really have a craving, I revert back to dairy based cheese.

I know this is not good for me and knowing this is important, as I limit what I consume to a very small amount, but I also try my best to counter act any negative effects that eating cheese may cause me. If I decide to eat cheese I make sure to eat extra leafy greens or other fruits and veggies and I make sure my water intake is greater than usual. This way I can at least help escort the cheese through my system as quickly as possible.

My other main exception is eating after my last meal of the day. Intermittent fasting has done wonders for me, but there are times when hunger seems to get the best of me, so I am faced with a dilemma. Do I sit and listen to my stomach growling and feel hungry or do I do something about it? Well, I've done both and I can assure you, allowing the stomach to growl and feel hungry all night is no fun! My solution? A simple exception.

If it is within a few hours of my last meal and I am feeling peckish, I will make some lightly salted popcorn. In order to ensure this is as healthy for me as possible, I do not make microwave popcorn. In fact, I haven't used a microwave in over a decade, but that is a whole different story! I make popcorn the old fashion way, in a pan on the stove top. If you have never made popcorn like this, you should try it!

The process is simple. Get some organic popcorn kernels, cooking oil (I use organic coconut oil) and a cooking pot with a lid. You may have to try a few times to get the amounts correct, but typically I will make a single layer of popcorn kernels in the bottom of the pan

NOTES:_____

_____

and then add enough oil to barely cover the kernels. Then put the lid on and turn on the heat. You don't need to do much after that, except to listen and give the pot a shake every now and then. Stove top popcorn making can be hazardous, as you are dealing with cooking oil and heat or open flame. Be very careful if you decide to try this method.

At some point the popcorn will start popping rapidly, when the popcorn starts popping less frequently remove it from the heat, so the kernels at the bottom do not burn. When taking the lid off be careful of steam that can come out. It can burn you if you're not careful. Pour the popcorn in a bowl and lightly salt. NO BUTTER!!! This is not for movie night, this is an eating habit exception, so use it the way it was intended, which is to help you along the way when you find yourself faced with a hunger hurdle.

These are really the only consistent exceptions I have in my eating habits. Every now and then I will break my own rules, but that is because I know what I'm doing and have expressed to myself the willingness to accept the consequences of my actions. For example, there is a restaurant that we go to which serves an amazing honey butter croissant. When we go to this restaurant, which is not very often, I will usually have one of these delights.

It's got lots more sugar than I usually eat and it is not gluten free, so I most likely will end up with a headache or joint pain as a result of eating it. But I know these things ahead of time, so I am completely aware of what I will be doing to myself. There have been times when I did not order them, as I just didn't feel up to dealing with the consequences. We have to be willing to police our own habits and make common sense choices, even when our taste buds are begging us to be bad!

NOTES:_____

_____

I will say this however, if I decide to eat something that I know will cause me an issue, I have no right to complain about my choice. Heck, I made the bad choice, so why should I complain about it? I actually have a saying about this, "If you hit yourself in the head with a hammer, don't complain about your headache!" This simply means if you make a choice that causes you an issue, keep quiet and deal with the issue you created. If I want that croissant that badly, then I have to be prepared to suffer the headache and suffer in silence. It is not appropriate to make others uncomfortable with my complaints, especially if it was something I chose to do to myself!

Health is really about balance, which is why I do not try to tell people to "cut everything bad out of your eating habits." This just wouldn't be realistic and is one of the main reasons people cannot stick to a "diet". Most diets require you to do things that you simply will not do, at least not forever. Instead of setting yourself up for failure, enter this journey with realistic expectations and create eating habits that benefit you the majority of the time. Then if you slip up or indulge every now and then, the ramifications will not be nearly as bad.

While it is important to establish exceptions to your eating habits, so you can deal with the realities you will be faced with, it is also important to limit those exceptions and stick to your healthy eating habits.

Eat right, stay hydrated by drinking plenty of good water, be active and remember that you deserve to feel good, be heathy and be happy. Embrace positive change and discover the New You!

NOTES:_____

_____

# DISCOVERING THE MAGIC PILL

You've reached the final page of the main body of this book and you should be very proud of yourself! You've taken an important step to making a positive change in your life, but there are still nearly 100 more pages of valuable information, so don't stop reading! Every page is important to your journey to health and happiness.

I hope while reading this book you have come to the conclusion that, contrary to what companies offering the latest and greatest lotions, potions or fad diets are saying and, even contrary to the title of this book, there is no actual "magic pill"! But don't be disappointed, because while there is no magic pill, in life, THERE IS MAGIC! You don't need to look for a pill to find the magic of health and happiness. In fact, the magic has been looking at you in the mirror your entire life.

You see, you hold the power of an unimaginable magic deep inside yourself. All you have to do is continue to take action, make the right lifestyle choices and embrace positive changes that work best for you. Like magic you can make those bothersome aches and pains subside; you can make your waist line shrink more and more; you can find the happiness you've always wanted; and maybe you can even add some precious time on this amazing place we all call home.

The magic is yours, so set your magic free and discover just how incredible your life can be.

### A "Magic Pill" doesn't exist!

### *THE MAGIC...IS YOU!*

141

NOTES:_____

_____

# GLOSSARY OF HEALTH BUZZ WORDS

This section is more than just a glossary of the hottest health related buzz words; it is also a reference guide to expand your health knowledge. They say "Knowledge is Power", but I disagree with this. Knowledge is POTENTIAL power, APPLIED knowledge is power! If you don't use the knowledge you have, then is it really empowering you? Of course not!

And on the flipside, you need to have the knowledge, because you can't use something you don't have! So, while you may not think you need to read all of the health related buzz words contained in this section, as some of them may not specifically apply to you or your situation, I would strongly suggest that you read them all anyway. You may discover some new information in this section, which will help you expand your own knowledge, even if what you've learned doesn't seem applicable to you; it may just help someone you know.

So let's take a look at what the health related buzzwords you keep hearing actually mean!

## ACIDIC

In the context of the human body, the term "acidic" refers to a substance that has a low pH, meaning it has a high concentration of hydrogen ions. In general, substances with a pH lower than 7 are considered acidic, while those with a pH higher than 7 are considered basic or alkaline. The pH scale ranges from 0 to 14, with 7 being neutral.

In the body, the pH of various fluids and tissues can vary significantly. For example, the pH of the stomach is typically around 2, which is highly acidic, while the pH

142

of the blood is around 7.4, which is slightly alkaline. The body has a number of mechanisms in place to maintain a stable pH, as deviations from the normal range can have serious consequences for health, including death.

In general, acidic substances can have a corrosive effect on tissues and may be harmful if consumed in large quantities. However, the body also uses acidity in certain processes, such as in the digestion of food and the immune system's response to infections.

## ALKALINE IONIZED WATER

Alkaline ionized water is water that has been subjected to an ionization process in order to increase its pH level and reduce its acidity. This process involves the use of an electrolysis machine, which passes an electric current through the water to separate it into alkaline and acidic components. The resulting alkaline water has a higher pH level than tap water, which means it is less acidic.

Proponents of alkaline ionized water claim that it has a number of health benefits, including improving hydration, balancing the body's pH level, and neutralizing harmful toxins in the body.

I personally use and recommend the water ionizers manufactured by Enagic®. If you decide to invest in a water ionizer, in order to start drinking alkaline ionized water, get your device from Enagic®, you'll be glad you did!

On a side note, bottled alkaline waters are not the same as the water produced when you have your own water ionizer, so don't be tricked by slick marketing and advertising trying to convince you otherwise.

143

NOTES:_____

_____

## ALKALINITY

Alkalinity refers to the ability of a substance to neutralize acids. In the human body, alkalinity is important for maintaining a healthy pH balance in the blood and other bodily fluids.

The pH scale measures the acidity or basicity (alkalinity) of a substance, with a range from 0 to 14. A substance with a pH of 7 is considered neutral, while a substance with a pH less than 7 is considered acidic, and a substance with a pH greater than 7 is considered basic or alkaline.

The pH of the human body is tightly regulated and is typically slightly alkaline, with a range of 7.35 to 7.45. This is because the body's cells and tissues function optimally within this pH range. If the pH of the body becomes too acidic or too alkaline, it can lead to serious health problems.

Maintaining the proper pH balance in the body is important for several reasons. First, it helps to ensure that enzymes and other proteins function properly. Enzymes are proteins that catalyze chemical reactions in the body, and they are sensitive to pH. If the pH of the body becomes too acidic or too alkaline, it can disrupt the activity of enzymes, which can lead to problems with metabolism and other processes.

Second, the pH of the body can affect the solubility of certain substances, such as minerals and electrolytes. For example, calcium, which is important for healthy bones and teeth, is more soluble at a slightly alkaline pH. If the pH becomes too acidic, calcium can be less soluble and may be excreted from the body, leading to a deficiency.

Finally, maintaining a healthy pH balance in the body is important for the immune system. The body's immune

144

cells are more effective at fighting off infections and diseases when the pH is slightly alkaline.

## ANTIOXIDANTS

Antioxidants are substances that can help protect cells in the body from damage caused by free radicals. Free radicals are unstable molecules that can damage cells and contribute to the development of various diseases, such as cancer and heart disease. Antioxidants work by neutralizing free radicals, which helps to prevent or repair damage to cells.

There are many different types of antioxidants, including vitamins, minerals, and phytochemicals (plant compounds). Some common antioxidant vitamins include vitamin A, vitamin C, and vitamin E. Minerals such as selenium and zinc also have antioxidant properties. Phytochemicals found in plant-based foods, such as lycopene in tomatoes and flavonoids in berries, are also believed to have antioxidant effects.

Antioxidants can be found in a variety of foods, including fruits, vegetables, whole grains, nuts, and seeds. Some examples of foods that are high in antioxidants include berries, leafy green vegetables, tomatoes, sweet potatoes, and nuts. It is important to get a variety of antioxidants through a healthy diet, as each type of antioxidant can provide different health benefits.

There is some evidence to suggest that antioxidant supplements may help to reduce the risk of certain diseases, but more research is needed to confirm this. In general, it is recommended to get antioxidants from a varied and healthy diet rather than relying on supplements.

NOTES:_____
_____

In summary, antioxidants are substances that can help protect cells from damage caused by free radicals. They can be found in a variety of foods, including fruits, vegetables, whole grains, nuts, and seeds. It is important to get a variety of antioxidants through a healthy diet, as each type can provide different health benefits. There is some evidence to suggest that antioxidant supplements may be helpful, but more research is needed to confirm this.

## ARTIFICIAL SWEETENER

Artificial sweeteners are substances that are used as a sugar substitute in food and beverages. They are typically much sweeter than sugar and are used to sweeten foods and beverages without adding calories or increasing the risk of tooth decay. Artificial sweeteners are often used by people who are trying to manage their weight, reduce their sugar intake, or control their blood sugar levels.

There are several types of artificial sweeteners available, including aspartame, sucralose, and stevia. Some people believe that artificial sweeteners may have potential health benefits, while others have concerns about their safety. It is important to note that the long-term effects of artificial sweeteners on human health are not fully understood and more research is needed to understand their potential risks and benefits.

There are several artificial sweeteners that are commonly used as substitutes for sugar in food and beverages. Here are a few examples:

1. Aspartame: This is a commonly used artificial sweetener that is found in a variety of products, including diet sodas, sugar-free gum, and low-calorie desserts. It is about 200 times sweeter

146

NOTES:_____

_____

than sugar and is usually used in combination with other sweeteners to improve the taste of low-calorie products.

2. Saccharin: This artificial sweetener is about 300-400 times sweeter than sugar and is commonly used in products such as diet sodas, sugar-free gum, and low-calorie desserts.

3. Sucralose: This sweetener is about 600 times sweeter than sugar and is commonly used in a variety of products, including diet sodas, sugar-free ice cream, and low-calorie baked goods.

4. Acesulfame potassium (Ace-K): This sweetener is about 200 times sweeter than sugar and is commonly used in a variety of products, including diet sodas, sugar-free gum, and low-calorie desserts.

5. Neotame: This sweetener is about 7,000-13,000 times sweeter than sugar and is commonly used in a variety of products, including diet sodas, sugar-free gum, and low-calorie desserts. It is similar to aspartame in chemical structure, but is more stable and longer lasting.

It's important to note that artificial sweeteners are not necessarily a healthy alternative to sugar, as they have been linked to a variety of health concerns, including weight gain, increased risk of diabetes, and other health problems. Some people may also experience side effects such as headaches or gastrointestinal issues after consuming artificial sweeteners.

## BIOAVAILABILITY

Bioavailability refers to the extent and rate at which a substance, such as a nutrient or medication, is

147

NOTES:_____

_____

absorbed and becomes available for use or storage in the body. It can be influenced by various factors, including the form in which the substance is taken, the presence of other substances that may interfere with its absorption, and individual differences in metabolism and digestion.

When it comes to nutrients, bioavailability can impact the body's ability to utilize the substance effectively. For example, the bioavailability of iron from plant sources is generally lower than that of iron from animal sources, due to the presence of compounds in plants that can inhibit iron absorption. Similarly, the bioavailability of certain nutrients, such as calcium and zinc, can be reduced by the presence of certain other substances, such as fiber.

In the case of medications, bioavailability refers to the amount of the drug that reaches the target site in the body and is able to produce the desired therapeutic effect. The bioavailability of a medication can be affected by various factors, including the way it is formulated (e.g. as a tablet or an injectable), the route of administration (e.g. oral, intravenous, or topical), and the presence of other substances that may interfere with its absorption or metabolism.

It is important to consider bioavailability when selecting a nutrient supplement or medication, as it can affect the effectiveness of the product. For example, a supplement with a high bioavailability may be more effective at improving nutrient status or treating a medical condition than a product with a lower bioavailability.

In summary, bioavailability is a key factor in determining the effectiveness of substances in the human body, and it is influenced by a variety of factors including the form in which the substance is taken, the presence of other

NOTES:_____

_____

substances that may interfere with its absorption, and individual differences in metabolism and digestion.

Bioavailability refers to the extent to which a nutrient or other substance is able to be absorbed and used by the body. Some factors that can affect the bioavailability of a substance include its chemical form, the presence of other substances that may inhibit or enhance its absorption, and the individual's digestive and metabolic functions.

Here are some examples of foods that are highly bioavailable:

- **Fruits and vegetables:** These are rich in vitamins, minerals, and other nutrients that are easily absorbed and used by the body.

- **Lean proteins:** Foods like chicken, fish, and tofu are high in protein and other nutrients that are easily absorbed and used by the body.

- **Whole grains:** These are a good source of complex carbohydrates, fiber, and other nutrients that are easily absorbed and used by the body.

On the other hand, some foods may not be as bioavailable due to their chemical form or the presence of other substances that inhibit absorption. For example:

- **Processed foods:** These often contain additives and preservatives that can interfere with the absorption of nutrients.

- **Foods high in phytates or oxalates:** These substances, found in some plant-based foods, can bind to minerals and prevent their absorption.

- **Foods high in fiber:** While fiber is important for good health, it can also reduce the absorption of some nutrients.

149

NOTES:_____

_____

It's important to note that the bioavailability of a nutrient can vary widely depending on the individual and their specific digestive and metabolic functions. Some people may absorb and use certain nutrients more efficiently than others.

## BLOOD SUGAR

Blood sugar, also known as blood glucose, is a type of sugar that is present in the blood and serves as the body's main source of energy. It is produced by the breakdown of carbohydrates in the diet and is regulated by hormones such as insulin and glucagon.

Normal blood sugar levels in adults are typically between 70 and 100 milligrams per deciliter (mg/dL) when fasting, and less than 140 mg/dL after eating. However, these levels can vary depending on age, sex, and other factors.

Elevated blood sugar levels, or hyperglycemia, can occur for a variety of reasons, including eating too many sugary or high-carbohydrate foods, not getting enough physical activity, and certain medical conditions such as diabetes. If left untreated, hyperglycemia can lead to serious health complications, such as heart disease, nerve damage, and kidney damage.

On the other hand, low blood sugar levels, or hypoglycemia, can also be dangerous. This can occur when the body's blood sugar levels drop too low, usually due to a missed meal, excessive exercise, or certain medications. Symptoms of hypoglycemia include dizziness, shakiness, and sweating. If left untreated, hypoglycemia can lead to seizures and loss of consciousness.

To maintain healthy blood sugar levels, it is important to eat a well-balanced diet that is low in added sugars and

NOTES:_____

_____

high in fiber. Getting regular physical activity, managing stress, and monitoring blood sugar levels can also help maintain healthy blood sugar levels. If you have a medical condition that affects your blood sugar levels, such as diabetes, it is important to work with a healthcare provider to develop a treatment plan that is right for you.

## BMI – BODY MASS INDEX

The body mass index (BMI) is a measure of body fat based on height and weight that is used to determine whether a person is underweight, normal weight, overweight, or obese. It is calculated by dividing a person's weight in kilograms by their height in meters squared.

The World Health Organization (WHO) has established the following categories for interpreting BMI:

- Underweight: BMI less than 18.5
- Normal weight: BMI between 18.5 and 24.9
- Overweight: BMI between 25 and 29.9
- Obese: BMI greater than or equal to 30

It's important to note that BMI is not a perfect measure of body fat and should not be used as the sole criteria for determining a person's health status. Other factors, such as muscle mass, bone density, and distribution of fat, can affect a person's BMI and should be considered when evaluating a person's overall health.

## BOTTLED WATER

The vast majority of bottled waters are simply reprocessed tap water; however, in some cases, it has

151

NOTES:_____

_____

not been reprocessed or filtered and is literally water from a public source being poured into a plastic container and sold for a premium price. In almost every situation tap water is cleaner, safer and less expensive, but not quite as convenient, which is really the only reason anyone would purchase bottled water. The bottled water industry has been under much scrutiny in the past decade for misleading advertising practices, disruption of natural water resources, environmental impact issues and potential health hazards created by chemicals in the plastic or even microscopic pieces of plastic actually ending up in the water being consumed.

Here are a few potential issues that may arise when consuming bottled water.

1. Contamination: Bottled water can potentially become contaminated with microorganisms or other impurities if it is not properly treated or handled. This can occur during the bottling process, or if the water is stored in unsanitary conditions.

2. Plastic leaching: The use of plastic bottles for storing water can lead to the leaching of chemicals from the plastic into the water, especially if the bottles are exposed to heat or sunlight. This can be a concern for some people, as the long-term effects of consuming these chemicals are not fully understood.

3. Cost: In some cases, bottled water can be more expensive than tap water, which can be a financial burden for some people.

Overall, it is important to purchase bottled water from reputable sources and to follow proper storage and handling guidelines to minimize the risk of contamination or other issues.

NOTES:_____

_____

It is difficult to quantify the number of contaminants that have been found in bottled water, as different brands and types of bottled water may contain different contaminants at different levels. Some common contaminants that have been found in bottled water include bacteria, minerals, and chemicals such as chlorine and fluoride. In addition, some studies have found that certain types of plastic bottles may leach chemicals into the water, which can also contribute to the presence of contaminants in the water.

It is important to note that all bottled water must meet certain safety standards set by regulatory agencies, such as the Food and Drug Administration (FDA) in the United States. However, these standards may not be as strict as those for tap water, and bottled water may still contain some contaminants. It is always a good idea to research the quality of the bottled water you are considering purchasing, and to consider alternative sources of drinking water if you have concerns about contaminants.

The environmental impact of bottled water can be significant.

First, the production of plastic bottles for water requires a significant amount of energy and resources, including oil and natural gas. The production and transportation of bottled water also generates greenhouse gas emissions, which contribute to climate change.

Additionally, the disposal of plastic bottles can be harmful to the environment. Many plastic bottles end up in landfills, where they can take hundreds of years to decompose. Some bottles end up as litter, which can be harmful to wildlife and the natural environment.

Finally, the transportation of bottled water can also have environmental impacts, as it requires fuel to transport the bottles to their final destination.

153

NOTES:_____

_____

Overall, the environmental impact of bottled water can be significant and reducing or eliminating the use of bottled water can help to reduce these impacts. Instead, consider using a reusable water bottle and filling it with tap water, which can be a more environmentally friendly option.

## CAFFEINE

Caffeine is a naturally occurring stimulant found in plants such as coffee, tea, cocoa beans, and other plants. It is also found in some medications and energy drinks. Caffeine works by stimulating the central nervous system, which can make you feel more awake and alert.

When caffeine is consumed, it is absorbed into the bloodstream and travels to the brain, where it blocks the action of a neurotransmitter called adenosine. This helps to increase the activity of other neurotransmitters such as dopamine and norepinephrine, which can improve mood and concentration.

Caffeine can have a range of effects on the body, including:

- Increased heart rate and blood pressure
- Increased alertness and energy
- Improved mood
- Improved concentration and memory
- Increased urine production

Here are some of the potential hazards of consuming caffeine:

1. Insomnia: Caffeine can interfere with the body's natural sleep-wake cycle, making it harder to fall asleep or stay asleep.

154

NOTES:_____
_____

2. Anxiety and restlessness: Caffeine can increase feelings of anxiety and nervousness, particularly in people who are sensitive to its effects.

3. Heart palpitations: Caffeine can cause heart palpitations, which are episodes of rapid or irregular heartbeat.

4. Dehydration: Caffeine can act as a diuretic, increasing urine production and leading to dehydration.

5. Dependence: Regular caffeine consumption can lead to physical dependence, resulting in withdrawal symptoms such as headache, fatigue, and irritability when caffeine intake is reduced or stopped.

It is generally recommended to limit caffeine intake to moderate levels, typically no more than 400 milligrams per day for adults. It is also important to pay attention to how your body reacts to caffeine and to be mindful of any negative effects it may have on your health.

## CALISTHENICS

Calisthenics is a form of exercise that uses your body weight and gravity as resistance to strengthen and tone your muscles. It typically involves performing a variety of exercises that use movements such as push-ups, squats, lunges, and planks, without the use of equipment or weights. Calisthenics exercises can be modified to accommodate different fitness levels and goals, making them a popular choice for people of all ages and abilities. Some people use calisthenics as a standalone workout, while others incorporate it into their fitness routine as a way to supplement other forms of exercise, such as running or weight lifting.

155

NOTES:_____

_____

## CARBOHYDRATES / CARBS

Carbohydrates are a type of macronutrient that are an important source of energy for the human body. They are found in a variety of foods, including grains, fruits, vegetables, and dairy products, and are composed of carbon, hydrogen, and oxygen atoms. When carbohydrates are consumed, they are broken down into simple sugars (such as glucose) in the body, which can be used for energy or stored for later use. There are different types of carbohydrates, including simple carbs (like those found in refined sugars and processed foods) and complex carbs (like those found in whole grains and legumes). The human body needs a certain amount of carbohydrates to function properly, but consuming too many can lead to weight gain and other health issues.

Carbohydrates are a type of nutrient found in many foods and are an important source of energy for the body. Here are some examples of common foods that contain carbohydrates:

1. Grains: bread, pasta, rice, oats, quinoa, and cereal
2. Starchy vegetables: potatoes, sweet potatoes, and winter squash
3. Legumes: beans, lentils, and peas
4. Fruits: apples, bananas, oranges, and berries
5. Milk and dairy products: milk, yogurt, and cheese
6. Snacks: chips, crackers, and cookies
7. Sugary foods and drinks: candy, soda, and fruit juice

It's important to note that not all carbohydrates are created equal, and some types of carbs may be more beneficial for health than others. For example, whole grains, legumes, and vegetables are generally

NOTES:_____

_____

considered healthier sources of carbs because they are rich in fiber and other nutrients, while sugary foods and drinks are often high in empty calories and can contribute to weight gain and other health problems if consumed in excess.

## CARDIO

Cardio, short for cardiovascular exercise, refers to physical activity that increases the heart rate and circulation. Cardio exercises can include activities like running, cycling, swimming, and walking. These exercises are beneficial for the body because they help to improve cardiovascular health by strengthening the heart and increasing blood flow. Cardio exercises can also help to improve lung function and increase endurance. They can also help to reduce the risk of heart disease, stroke, and other health conditions. In addition, cardio exercise can help to improve mental health by reducing stress and improving mood. It is generally recommended that adults engage in at least 150 minutes of moderate intensity cardio exercise per week, or 75 minutes of vigorous intensity cardio exercise, in order to maintain good health.

## CHEAT DAY

A cheat day is a day where you allow yourself to eat foods that you normally would not eat as part of your regular diet. People often have cheat days as a way to indulge in their favorite foods or to give themselves a break from their usual healthy eating habits. Some people plan cheat days as part of a diet or weight loss plan, while others may just have a cheat day spontaneously whenever they feel like it. It's important to note that while having a cheat day can be a fun and

NOTES:_____

_____

enjoyable way to relax your diet, it's important to be mindful of your overall food intake and to make sure that your cheat day doesn't turn into a habit that undermines your healthy eating habits.

It is extremely important to limit your cheat days! Many people start with a cheat day that turns into a cheat week, month, year or even decade. The most important word in the term "cheat day" is "cheat", as the truth of the matter is that the only person really being cheated on a cheat day is the person doing the cheating. While treating yourself to a cheat day may allow you to justify indulging in a food that you know is not good for you, what you are actually doing is cheating yourself of good health and setting yourself up for possible problems. Just like anything in life, cheating has its consequences, so if you cannot completely eliminate cheat days, at least limit them to as few as possible, your health and happiness will thank you!

## CHEMICAL FREE

The term "chemical free" as it pertains to food is often used to describe products that do not contain any synthetic or artificial chemicals or ingredients. However, it is important to note that all food contains chemicals, as chemicals are present in all substances, including natural ones.

For example, water is a chemical made up of hydrogen and oxygen atoms, and fruits and vegetables contain a variety of chemicals such as vitamins, minerals, and phytochemicals that are essential for good health.

Therefore, it is not accurate to describe any food as being completely "chemical free." Instead, the term is often used to imply that a food or product is made with

NOTES:_____

_____

natural, whole ingredients and does not contain any synthetic or artificial chemicals or additives.

It is important to be aware that the use of the term "chemical free" on food labels is not regulated, and it is up to the manufacturer to determine how they want to use the term. It is always a good idea to carefully read labels and do research to understand the ingredients in the products you are purchasing.

## CHOLESTEROL

Cholesterol is a type of fat (lipid) that is produced by the liver and found in certain foods. It is an important part of the structure of cell membranes and is used to produce hormones, vitamin D, and bile acids, which help to digest fat.

There are two main types of cholesterol:

1. Low-density lipoprotein (LDL) cholesterol: This is often referred to as "bad" cholesterol because high levels of LDL cholesterol in the blood can increase the risk of heart disease.

2. High-density lipoprotein (HDL) cholesterol: This is often referred to as "good" cholesterol because high levels of HDL cholesterol in the blood can help to protect against heart disease.

In general, it is important to maintain a healthy balance of cholesterol in the body. This can be achieved through a healthy diet, regular physical activity, and, in some cases, medication. If you have questions about your cholesterol levels or how to manage them, it is important to speak with a healthcare provider.

Cholesterol is a type of fat that is found in the bloodstream and in all of your body's cells. It is

159

NOTES:_____

_____

necessary for the proper functioning of the body, but too much cholesterol can be harmful.

There are two main types of cholesterol: high-density lipoprotein (HDL) cholesterol and low-density lipoprotein (LDL) cholesterol.

HDL cholesterol is often referred to as "good" cholesterol because it helps remove excess cholesterol from the body. High levels of HDL cholesterol are associated with a lower risk of heart disease.

LDL cholesterol is often referred to as "bad" cholesterol because it can build up in the walls of the arteries, leading to a condition called atherosclerosis. Atherosclerosis is a leading cause of heart attacks and strokes. High levels of LDL cholesterol are associated with an increased risk of heart disease.

It is important to maintain a healthy balance of good and bad cholesterol in order to reduce the risk of heart disease and other health problems. This can be achieved through a healthy diet, regular exercise, and in some cases, medication.

There are no specific foods that can lower or raise cholesterol levels. However, certain foods may have an impact on cholesterol levels. For example, foods that are high in saturated and trans fats, such as fried foods, processed foods, and unhealthy fats (like butter and lard) can increase LDL cholesterol levels. On the other hand, foods that are high in fiber, such as oats, beans, fruits, and vegetables, may help to lower LDL cholesterol levels.

It's important to maintain a healthy and balanced diet, including a variety of fruits, vegetables, whole grains, lean proteins, and healthy fats, as part of a overall healthy lifestyle to help maintain healthy cholesterol levels. It's also important to exercise regularly and avoid tobacco products, which can also have an impact on

NOTES:_____

cholesterol levels. If you have concerns about your cholesterol levels or your risk for heart disease, it's a good idea to speak with a healthcare professional.

## CHRONIC

In medicine, the term "chronic" refers to a condition or disease that persists or progresses over a long period of time. Chronic conditions are typically characterized by their duration, which is often measured in months or years. Examples of chronic conditions include diabetes, high blood pressure, heart disease, and certain types of cancer. These conditions typically require ongoing medical treatment and management in order to prevent or minimize their impact on the individual's health. Chronic conditions can often be managed effectively through a combination of lifestyle changes, such as diet and exercise, and medical therapies, such as medications or surgery.

There are many chronic health conditions that can affect people of all ages. Some examples include:

1. Asthma: a respiratory condition that causes difficulty breathing and can be triggered by various factors, such as exercise, allergies, and pollution.

2. Diabetes: a condition in which the body is unable to properly use and store glucose, a type of sugar, resulting in high blood sugar levels.

3. Heart disease: a group of conditions that affect the heart and can lead to heart attacks and stroke.

4. High blood pressure: a condition in which the blood vessels have persistently high pressure, which can increase the risk of heart attack, stroke, and other serious health problems.

NOTES:_____

_____

5. Cancer: a group of diseases characterized by the uncontrolled growth and spread of abnormal cells in the body.

6. Chronic obstructive pulmonary disease (COPD): a lung disease that makes it difficult to breathe and can be caused by smoking or exposure to other toxins.

7. Arthritis: a group of conditions that cause inflammation in the joints, leading to pain and stiffness.

8. Multiple sclerosis (MS): a condition that affects the central nervous system and can cause muscle weakness, difficulty with balance and coordination, and vision problems.

9. Depression: a mental health disorder characterized by persistent feelings of sadness and hopelessness.

10. Chronic kidney disease: a condition in which the kidneys are damaged and unable to filter waste and excess fluids from the body effectively.

This is not an exhaustive list, as there are many other chronic health conditions that can affect people. It is important to seek medical advice if you are experiencing any ongoing health concerns.

## CLEAN EATING

Clean eating is a term that refers to a style of eating that focuses on whole, minimally processed foods. It involves choosing foods that are as close to their natural state as possible and avoiding processed, refined, and artificial ingredients. Clean eating often includes an emphasis on fresh fruits and vegetables, whole grains, lean proteins, and healthy fats, and may

NOTES:_____

exclude certain types of food and ingredients, such as added sugars, refined grains, and unhealthy fats. The goal of clean eating is to nourish the body with nutrient-dense foods that support overall health and wellness.

## DEGENERATIVE DISEASE

A degenerative disease is a type of medical condition that progressively worsens over time. This can refer to a wide range of conditions that affect different parts of the body, including the brain, nerves, muscles, bones, and organs. Degenerative diseases often result in the loss of function or structure in the affected body parts, and they can be caused by a variety of factors such as genetics, age, lifestyle, and environmental exposures. Some examples of degenerative diseases include Alzheimer's disease, Parkinson's disease, osteoarthritis, and heart disease. Degenerative diseases are often chronic conditions that require ongoing medical management and can significantly impact a person's quality of life.

## DEHYDRATION

Dehydration is a condition in which the body lacks sufficient fluids to function properly. It occurs when the body loses more fluids than it takes in, either through sweating, vomiting, diarrhea, or other means. When the body is dehydrated, it can lead to symptoms such as thirst, fatigue, dizziness, dry mouth, and dark urine. Severe dehydration can cause more serious symptoms, such as fainting, rapid heartbeat, and confusion.

Dehydration can be dangerous, especially in young children and older adults, and can lead to serious health problems if left untreated. To prevent dehydration, it is important to drink plenty of fluids, particularly water,

NOTES:_____

_____

and to replace fluids lost through sweating and other means.

Dehydration can cause a range of health issues, including:

1. Dry mouth and thirst: When your body is dehydrated, you may experience dry mouth and a constant feeling of thirst.

2. Headache: Dehydration can cause a headache, especially if you are prone to migraines.

3. Fatigue: Dehydration can lead to fatigue, as the body lacks the fluids it needs to function properly.

4. Dizziness: Dehydration can cause dizziness, especially if you are standing up or moving around quickly.

5. Dry skin: Dehydration can cause dry, flaky skin and can exacerbate existing skin conditions such as eczema.

6. Constipation: Dehydration can cause constipation, as the body lacks the fluids needed to soften and move waste through the intestines.

7. Muscle cramps: Dehydration can cause muscle cramps, especially in the legs and feet.

8. Heat stroke: In extreme cases, dehydration can lead to heat stroke, which is a serious and potentially life-threatening condition.

Darkly colored pee can be a sign of dehydration. It can also be attributed to other issues, so if your pee appears as a dark yellow or even brown, you may want to consult with your physician. When you are properly hydrated your pee should be clear or have a light tint of yellow, so use this as a way to monitor your hydration. If you take supplements, your pee may be darker yellow,

NOTES:_____

_____

which could be a sign that the supplements are not being absorbed or utilized.

In severe cases, dehydration can lead to more serious health issues, such as kidney failure, seizures, and coma. It is important to drink enough fluids, especially when it is hot or you are engaging in physical activity. In my opinion alkaline ionized water is the best choice for proper hydration. If you are concerned about your hydration status or have symptoms of dehydration, it is important to speak with a healthcare provider for proper evaluation and treatment...and drink more water!

## DETOX

Detox refers to the process of eliminating toxins from the body. Toxins are substances that can be harmful to the body and can come from a variety of sources, including the environment, food, and lifestyle habits. Detoxing can involve a variety of methods, such as drinking plenty of water, exercising, eating a healthy diet, and taking supplements to support the body's natural detoxification processes.

Some people also use detox programs or cleanses that involve cutting out certain foods or beverages or following a specific diet plan in an effort to remove toxins from the body. While the body has its own natural detoxification systems, such as the liver, kidneys, and lymphatic system, some people believe that undergoing a detox can improve their overall health and well-being. However, it is important to consult a healthcare professional before starting a detox program, as some methods may not be safe or appropriate for everyone.

There are many different ways to detox the human body, but it's important to note that the term "detox" can be

165

NOTES:_____

_____

misleading and is often used to promote products or practices that have little to no scientific basis. The body is already equipped with organs (such as the liver and kidneys) that are responsible for filtering out toxins and waste products, so it's generally not necessary to "detox" in the way that the term is often used. That being said, there are several things that you can do to support the body's natural detoxification processes:

1. **Eat a healthy diet:** A diet that is rich in fruits, vegetables, and whole grains can provide the nutrients that the body needs to function properly and support the detoxification process.

2. **Stay hydrated:** Drinking plenty of water can help to flush toxins out of the body and keep the kidneys functioning properly.

3. **Exercise regularly:** Regular physical activity can help to improve circulation, which can help to move toxins through the body more effectively.

4. **Get plenty of sleep:** Adequate sleep is important for overall health, and it can also help the body to repair and regenerate itself.

5. **Avoid unhealthy habits:** Smoking, excessive alcohol consumption, and drug abuse can all put additional strain on the body's detoxification systems. Limiting or eliminating these habits can support the body's natural detoxification processes.

6. **Consider natural remedies:** Some people may choose to use natural remedies, such as herbal teas or supplements, to support the body's detoxification processes. It's important to speak with a healthcare provider before using any natural remedies, as they can sometimes interact with medications or have other risks.

166

# DIABETES

Diabetes is a chronic condition characterized by high levels of sugar (glucose) in the blood. There are two main types of diabetes: type 1 and type 2.

Type 1 diabetes, also known as insulin-dependent diabetes, is caused by the body's inability to produce insulin. Insulin is a hormone produced by the pancreas that helps regulate the amount of sugar in the blood. People with type 1 diabetes must take insulin injections or use an insulin pump to manage their blood sugar levels.

Type 2 diabetes, also known as non-insulin dependent diabetes, is caused by the body's inability to properly use insulin. People with type 2 diabetes may be able to manage their condition with lifestyle changes, such as diet and exercise, or with oral medications. However, some people with type 2 diabetes may also need insulin injections.

Both types of diabetes can lead to serious complications if left untreated, including heart disease, stroke, kidney damage, and nerve damage. Managing diabetes involves regularly monitoring blood sugar levels, following a healthy diet, and getting regular physical activity.

There is no "cure" for diabetes, but it can be managed effectively with proper diet, treatment and care. It is important for people with diabetes to assume personal responsibility for their actions that either improve or worsen their diabetes and they should work closely with their healthcare team to develop a treatment plan that works for them.

NOTES:_____

_____

## ELECTROLYTES

Electrolytes are substances that contain ions and can conduct electricity when dissolved in water. They play a crucial role in many biological processes, including maintaining the balance of fluids in the body, transmitting nerve impulses, and contracting muscles.

There are several types of electrolytes, including sodium, potassium, calcium, and chlorine. These ions can be found in various foods and beverages, and they can also be obtained through electrolyte supplements.

Sodium is an electrolyte that helps regulate the balance of fluids in the body and is important for maintaining normal blood pressure. It can be found in foods such as salt, soy sauce, and processed foods. Potassium is another electrolyte that helps regulate heart function and muscle contractions. It can be found in foods such as bananas, potatoes, and avocados.

Calcium is an electrolyte that is important for building and maintaining strong bones and teeth. It also plays a role in nerve and muscle function. Good sources of calcium include dairy products, leafy green vegetables, and nuts. Chlorine is an electrolyte that helps maintain the balance of fluids in the body and is important for digestion. It can be found in foods such as salt and processed foods.

Electrolyte imbalances can occur when the body loses too much fluid or when the levels of electrolytes in the body become imbalanced. This can be caused by factors such as illness, diarrhea, vomiting, or excessive sweating. Symptoms of an electrolyte imbalance can include fatigue, muscle weakness, cramps, and irregular heartbeat.

It is important to maintain proper electrolyte balance by consuming a healthy and balanced diet and drinking

NOTES:_____

enough fluids. In some cases, electrolyte supplements may be necessary to restore balance. It is important to speak with a healthcare provider if you are concerned about your electrolyte levels or if you are experiencing symptoms of an electrolyte imbalance.

## ENERGY

In the context of the human body, energy refers to the capacity to do work or produce change. It is the driving force behind all physical and physiological processes in the body. The body uses energy to perform various functions, such as maintaining body temperature, contracting muscles, and supporting various metabolic processes.

The body obtains energy from the food we eat, which is converted into a form of energy called ATP (adenosine triphosphate). ATP is used by cells to power various chemical reactions and processes. The body's energy needs vary depending on a person's age, sex, weight, and level of physical activity.

In addition to the energy used by the body to perform physiological functions, the body also requires energy for mental activities, such as thinking, learning, and decision-making. This energy is provided by the brain's metabolism, which is fueled by a constant supply of glucose and oxygen.

Overall, energy is essential for the proper functioning of the human body and plays a vital role in maintaining health and well-being.

NOTES:_____

_____

## ESSENTIAL MINERALS

Essential minerals are substances that are necessary for the proper functioning of the human body. These minerals cannot be synthesized by the body and must be obtained from the diet or from supplements. There are six essential minerals that are required in large amounts by the body: calcium, chloride, magnesium, phosphorus, potassium, and sodium.

There are also trace minerals that are required in smaller amounts, including iron, copper, iodine, zinc, and selenium. These minerals are involved in a wide variety of important physiological processes, including the formation of bones and teeth, the regulation of fluid balance and blood pressure, and the synthesis of hormones and enzymes.

## EXERCISE

Exercise is any physical activity that helps to improve or maintain physical fitness and overall health. It can involve a wide range of activities, from low-intensity activities such as walking or stretching to high-intensity activities such as running or weightlifting.

Regular exercise can help to improve cardiovascular health, increase strength and flexibility, and reduce the risk of chronic diseases such as obesity, diabetes, and heart disease. It can also help to improve mental health and well-being by reducing stress and improving mood. It is important to find an exercise routine that is enjoyable and that can be easily incorporated into a person's daily routine.

NOTES:_____
_____

## FAD DIET

A fad diet is a diet that becomes popular for a short period of time, often because it claims to offer rapid weight loss or other health benefits. However, these diets are often not based on sound scientific principles and may not provide long-term results.

Fad diets may also be unhealthy, as they may exclude important nutrients or rely on a limited number of foods. It is generally not recommended to follow a fad diet, as a healthy, balanced diet that includes a variety of nutrient-rich foods is a better option for sustained weight loss and overall health. It is important to speak with a healthcare provider or a registered dietitian before starting any new diet.

Here are some examples of fad diets:

1. **The Atkins Diet:** This diet involves restricting carbohydrates and increasing the intake of fats and proteins. It is based on the idea that limiting carbs can help with weight loss and improve health markers.

2. **The South Beach Diet:** This diet is similar to the Atkins Diet, but it emphasizes the intake of "good" carbs and fats. It is marketed as a way to improve heart health and lose weight.

3. **The Keto Diet:** This diet involves drastically reducing the intake of carbs and increasing the intake of fats. It is based on the idea that this will put the body into a state of ketosis, where it burns fat for energy instead of carbs.

4. **The Paleolithic Diet:** This diet is based on the idea of eating like our ancestors did during the Paleolithic era, which means eating a lot of meat,

171

NOTES:_____

_____

vegetables, and fruits, and avoiding processed foods.

5. **The Raw Food Diet:** This diet involves eating only raw, uncooked foods, or foods that are cooked at a low temperature. It is based on the idea that cooking destroys nutrients and enzymes in food.

It's important to note that while some of these diets may lead to short-term weight loss, they are not necessarily healthy or sustainable in the long term. It's always a good idea to speak with a healthcare professional before starting any new diet or exercise program.

## FAST FOOD

Fast food is a type of food that is prepared and served quickly, typically at a fast food restaurant or drive-through. Fast food is typically less expensive and more convenient than other types of restaurant food, and is often high in calories, fat, and sugar. Examples of fast food include hamburgers, fries, chicken nuggets, pizza, and soft drinks.

Eating too much fast food can have serious health consequences. Fast food is often high in calories, fat, and added sugars, and can contribute to weight gain and obesity. It is also often high in sodium, which can lead to high blood pressure and an increased risk of stroke and heart disease.

In addition to the risks associated with the nutrients found in fast food, the preparation of fast food can also pose hazards. Many fast food items are fried, which can increase the risk of heart disease and other health problems. The use of preservatives and other chemicals in fast food can also be a concern, as they may have negative effects on the body over time.

172

Eating fast food regularly can also have negative impacts on mental health. Studies have shown that a diet high in fast food is associated with an increased risk of depression and other mental health problems. This may be due, in part, to the fact that fast food is often high in refined carbohydrates and low in nutrients that are important for brain health, such as omega-3 fatty acids and antioxidants.

It is important to limit the amount of fast food that you eat and to choose healthier options when possible. Instead of relying on fast food, it is better to prepare meals at home using fresh, whole ingredients. This will help you to maintain a healthy weight and reduce your risk of developing health problems associated with a diet high in fast food.

## FITNESS

Fitness refers to the ability of the human body to function effectively and efficiently in various physical activities and daily tasks. It is a measure of an individual's physical health and well-being, and it can be influenced by various factors such as genetics, diet, exercise, and overall lifestyle.

There are several components of physical fitness that are important for overall health, including:

1. Cardiorespiratory endurance: The ability of the heart, lungs, and blood vessels to deliver oxygen and nutrients to the body's tissues during sustained physical activity.

2. Muscular strength: The ability of muscles to exert force during physical activity.

3. Muscular endurance: The ability of muscles to perform repeated contractions or to continue

173

NOTES:_____

_____

functioning for an extended period of time without becoming tired.

4. Flexibility: The ability to move joints through their full range of motion.

5. Body composition: The ratio of fat to lean mass in the body.

Maintaining good physical fitness can help to reduce the risk of developing chronic health conditions such as obesity, heart disease, and type 2 diabetes, and it can also improve mental health and overall quality of life.

## GMO – GENETICALLY MODIFIED

GMO stands for genetically modified organism. A GMO is an organism that has been genetically modified in a laboratory using genetic engineering techniques. This means that the DNA of the organism has been altered in some way, either by adding, deleting, or changing the genetic material.

GMOs are created for a variety of purposes, including improving crop yields, increasing the nutritional value of food, and making plants more resistant to pests and diseases. Some common examples of GMOs include corn, soybeans, and cotton that have been genetically modified to be resistant to pests or herbicides.

There is ongoing debate about the safety and potential risks of GMOs. Some people are concerned about the potential negative impacts on the environment and on human health, while others believe that GMOs can help to address global food security and environmental challenges.

NOTES:_____

# HAPPINESS

Happiness is a feeling that is often sought after by many people. It is a feeling of contentment, joy, and satisfaction that can bring a sense of well-being and fulfillment to our lives. There are many factors that can contribute to our happiness, including our relationships, our work, and our overall sense of purpose and meaning.

One of the main reasons why being happy is important is that it can have a positive impact on our physical and mental health. Studies have shown that people who are happier tend to have lower rates of stress and anxiety, as well as a stronger immune system and lower risk of developing certain diseases. Happiness can also improve our mental health and overall well-being by helping us to feel more positive and optimistic about the future.

In addition to the physical and mental health benefits of happiness, it can also have a positive impact on our relationships and social connections. When we are happy, we are more likely to be kind, compassionate, and empathetic towards others, which can lead to stronger and more meaningful relationships.

Being happy can also have a positive impact on our work and productivity. People who are happy tend to be more motivated, focused, and productive, which can lead to greater success and fulfillment in their careers.

Overall, the importance of being happy cannot be overstated. It can have a positive impact on our physical and mental health, our relationships, and our work. It is something that we should all strive for and cultivate in our lives.

NOTES:_____

_____

## HEALTH

Health refers to the overall physical, mental, and social well-being of a person. In the context of the human body, health refers to the absence of disease or injury and the presence of physical and mental vitality. Good health allows a person to participate in the activities of daily living and to pursue their goals and objectives. It is important to maintain good health through proper nutrition, exercise, and other self-care practices, as well as seeking medical care when necessary. Health is not just the absence of disease, but also the presence of physical, mental, and social well-being.

## HEALTHY WEIGHT RANGE

Healthy weight range is a range of body weight that is considered optimal for good health. It is determined by various factors such as age, sex, height, and body composition. The healthy weight range is usually defined as a body mass index (BMI) between 18.5 and 24.9. However, it's important to note that BMI is not a perfect measure of health and other factors such as muscle mass and body fat percentage should also be considered.

Most people do not calculate their BMI, so finding your own healthy weight range in pounds is usually easier to figure out. This range typically has a variance of approximately twenty pounds, but your individual range doesn't need to fluctuate that much. I discovered that my ideal healthy weight range is between 190 – 200 pounds. At this weight I am happy with both how I feel and how I look.

NOTES:_____
_____

# HIGH FRUCTOSE CORN SYRUP

High fructose corn syrup (HFCS) is a sweetener that is commonly used in a variety of processed foods and beverages. It is made from corn starch that has been processed to increase the fructose content. HFCS is used as a sweetener because it is cheap, easy to transport, and blends well with other ingredients. It has a similar sweetness to sucrose (table sugar), but is often used in place of sugar in processed foods because it is less expensive and easier to blend into products.

HFCS has been the subject of controversy in recent years due to concerns about its potential health effects. Some studies have suggested that HFCS may contribute to the development of obesity and other health problems, although more research is needed to confirm these findings. Overall, it is recommended to limit your intake of added sugars, including HFCS, as part of a healthy diet.

High fructose corn syrup (HFCS) is a sweetener that is commonly used in processed foods and beverages. Some examples of foods that may contain high fructose corn syrup include:

1. Soft drinks and other sweetened beverages
2. Fruit drinks and sports drinks
3. Processed and packaged baked goods such as cookies, cakes, and pastries
4. Frozen desserts and ice cream
5. Candies and other sweets
6. Breakfast cereals
7. Condiments such as ketchup and salad dressing
8. Canned and packaged fruit
9. Packaged soups and sauces

NOTES:_____

_____

It's important to note that high fructose corn syrup is not found in all of these types of foods, and the amount of HFCS in a particular product may vary. Some food manufacturers have started to use alternative sweeteners in their products, so it's always a good idea to check the ingredient list on the packaging to see if HFCS is present.

## HOLISTIC

Holistic refers to the idea that the different parts of the human body, such as the physical, mental, and emotional aspects, are all interconnected and influence one another. In a holistic approach to healthcare, the focus is on treating the whole person, rather than just the symptoms of a particular condition or disorder. This can involve considering a person's lifestyle, diet, and other factors that may impact their overall health and well-being. Holistic practices often involve a variety of different treatments and therapies, such as herbal medicine, acupuncture, and meditation, in addition to more traditional Western medical approaches. The goal is to achieve balance and harmony within the body and mind, and to promote overall health and well-being.

## HYDRATION

Hydration is extremely important for maintaining the overall health and well-being of the human body. Water is essential for many vital functions in the body, including regulating body temperature, carrying nutrients to cells, and maintaining the balance of bodily fluids. When the body is properly hydrated, it is better able to perform these functions and maintain optimal health.

NOTES:_____
_____

One of the most obvious signs of dehydration is thirst, but there are other signs to look out for as well. These can include dry mouth, fatigue, headache, dizziness, and dark yellow urine. It is important to pay attention to these signs and take action to rehydrate as soon as possible.

There are many factors that can contribute to dehydration, including heat exposure, physical activity, and illness. It is especially important to stay hydrated in hot or humid environments, as the body sweats to regulate its temperature and can lose a significant amount of water. Similarly, during physical activity, the body sweats to cool down and can lose a lot of fluids. It is important to drink plenty of fluids before, during, and after exercise to replace any fluids lost through sweat.

Illness can also cause dehydration, especially if the person has a fever, diarrhea, or vomiting. It is important to drink plenty of fluids and replace electrolytes (such as sodium and potassium) lost through these processes.

Proper hydration is important for everyone, but it is especially crucial for certain groups of people, such as young children, the elderly, and athletes. Children and the elderly may be more susceptible to dehydration due to their smaller body size and potential for underlying health conditions. Athletes may also be at a higher risk for dehydration due to the demands of their sport and the amount of sweat they lose during training and competition.

In conclusion, hydration is essential for maintaining optimal health and well-being. It is important to pay attention to the signs of dehydration and take action to rehydrate as needed, especially in hot or humid environments, during physical activity, and when experiencing illness. Proper hydration is especially

NOTES:_____

_____

important for certain groups of people, including young children, the elderly, and athletes.

## HYPERTENSION

Hypertension, also known as high blood pressure, is a medical condition in which the blood pressure in the arteries is consistently elevated. Blood pressure is the force of blood pushing against the walls of the arteries as the heart pumps it around the body. Normal blood pressure is generally considered to be a reading of less than 120/80 mmHg (millimeters of mercury). Blood pressure readings above 140/90 mmHg are considered to be high, and readings above 180/120 mmHg are considered to be very high.

Hypertension is a serious condition because it can increase the risk of various health problems, including heart disease, stroke, kidney disease, and vision loss. It can also contribute to the development of other medical conditions, such as diabetes. While there is no cure for hypertension, it can be effectively managed through lifestyle changes, such as eating a healthy diet, getting regular exercise, and avoiding tobacco and excessive alcohol consumption, and through the use of medications as prescribed by a healthcare provider.

## IMMUNE SYSTEM

The immune system is a complex network of cells, tissues, and organs that work together to defend the body against attacks by foreign invaders, such as viruses and bacteria. It is a vital part of the body's defense mechanism and plays a crucial role in maintaining health and preventing diseases.

180

NOTES:_____

_____

The immune system is made up of several different types of cells, including white blood cells (also known as leukocytes) and antibodies, which are proteins produced by certain cells in response to the presence of a foreign substance (antigen) in the body. These cells and antibodies work together to recognize and attack foreign invaders, either directly (by killing them) or indirectly (by signaling other cells to do so).

The immune system also includes various organs and tissues that play a role in the immune response, such as the spleen, lymph nodes, and bone marrow. Overall, the immune system helps to protect the body from illness and disease by identifying and eliminating harmful substances and foreign invaders.

A compromised immune system refers to a condition in which the body's immune system is not functioning properly. The immune system is a complex network of cells, tissues, and organs that work together to defend the body against foreign invaders, such as bacteria, viruses, and toxins. When the immune system is compromised, it may not be able to effectively protect the body against these harmful substances, which can lead to an increased risk of illness and infection. There are many different factors that can compromise the immune system, including chronic stress, malnutrition, certain medications, and certain medical conditions such as HIV/AIDS or cancer.

An immune deficiency occurs when the immune system is not functioning properly. This can be due to a variety of reasons, including genetics, certain medications, and certain medical conditions. People with immune deficiencies may have a higher risk of infections and other health problems, as their bodies are not able to effectively fight off disease and infection. There are

181

several different types of immune deficiencies, including primary immune deficiencies, which are present from birth, and secondary immune deficiencies, which occur as a result of another medical condition or treatment. If you have an immune deficiency, it is important to work with a healthcare provider to manage your condition and reduce your risk of infections and other health problems.

## LIFESTYLE CHOICES

Lifestyle choices refer to the decisions that individuals make about how they live their lives, including their daily routines, habits, and activities. These choices can encompass a wide range of areas, including work, relationships, leisure activities, diet, exercise, and personal growth. Lifestyle choices can have a significant impact on an individual's overall well-being and quality of life, and are often influenced by personal values, goals, and circumstances. Some people may prioritize health and wellness in their lifestyle choices, while others may focus on career advancement or financial stability. Ultimately, lifestyle choices reflect the values and priorities of each individual and can change over time as people's goals and circumstances evolve.

The lifestyle choices a person makes relates directly to their level of personal responsibility. Personal responsibility is the concept that individuals are accountable for their own actions and decisions. It involves being responsible for one's own behavior and the consequences of that behavior, as well as making decisions and taking ownership of their own lives.

Personal responsibility requires individuals to take control of their own lives and make decisions that align with their values and goals. It also involves being accountable for the impact of those decisions on others

NOTES:_____
_____

and the larger community. Personal responsibility is an important aspect of personal development and can contribute to a sense of purpose, self-worth, and accomplishment.

While it is much easier to place the blame for our misgivings on others or situations outside of our control, the harsh reality is that the majority of the outcomes in our lives, good or bad, are a direct result of the choices we make. Assumption of personal responsibility for our lifestyle choices is one of the most important things we can do if we want to live a happy and healthy life!

## LOW-CARB DIET

Low carbohydrate diets are dietary approaches that involve limiting the intake of carbohydrates, typically in the form of sugars and starches, in order to promote weight loss and improve health. These diets are based on the idea that reducing carbohydrate intake can lead to a reduction in body weight, blood sugar levels, and other markers of health.

There are several different types of low carbohydrate diets, including the ketogenic diet, the Atkins diet, and the paleo diet. These diets vary in the amount of carbohydrates that are allowed and the types of foods that are emphasized.

The ketogenic diet, also known as the "keto" diet, is a very low carbohydrate diet that is high in fat. This diet involves restricting carbohydrate intake to less than 50 grams per day and replacing them with high-fat foods, such as meats, dairy products, and certain oils. The goal of the keto diet is to put the body into a state of ketosis, in which it begins to burn fat for energy rather than glucose. This diet has been shown to be effective for

183

weight loss and has been used to treat certain medical conditions, such as epilepsy.

The Atkins diet is a low carbohydrate diet that was developed by Dr. Robert Atkins in the 1970s. This diet involves gradually increasing the amount of carbohydrates allowed as weight loss progresses. The Atkins diet emphasizes protein-rich foods, such as meats and dairy products, and allows for the consumption of fats and some carbohydrates, such as vegetables and nuts.

## MALNOURISHED

Malnourished refers to a condition in which the body is not getting sufficient nutrients to support proper growth and function. This can be due to a variety of factors, including an inadequate diet, an inability to absorb nutrients due to a medical condition or medication, or an increased need for nutrients due to illness or physical stress. Malnutrition can lead to a wide range of health problems, including weakness, fatigue, impaired immune function, and an increased risk of infections and diseases. It is important to maintain a healthy, balanced diet and to seek medical attention if you are concerned about malnutrition.

## MEDICAL DEPENDENCY

Medical dependency refers to the reliance on medications or medical treatments to maintain health or manage a medical condition. This can include prescription medications, over-the-counter drugs, and other medical treatments such as therapies or surgeries.

There are many different types of medical conditions that can lead to dependency on medications or other

NOTES:_____

treatments. For example, individuals with chronic conditions such as diabetes or high blood pressure may require lifelong treatment with medications to manage their symptoms and prevent complications. Others may develop a dependency on pain medications following an injury or surgery, or may require medication to manage mental health conditions such as anxiety or depression.

Medical dependency can have both positive and negative impacts on an individual's health and quality of life. On the positive side, medications and other medical treatments can be essential for managing and improving the symptoms of many medical conditions. They can help individuals lead active and productive lives, and may even save lives in cases of severe or life-threatening conditions.

However, there can also be negative consequences of medical dependency. Some medications can have side effects that can affect an individual's quality of life or lead to other health problems. In some cases, individuals may become physically or psychologically dependent on certain medications, leading to difficulties when trying to stop or reduce their use. In addition, the cost of medications and other medical treatments can be a burden for many individuals, particularly those without insurance or with limited coverage.

It is important for individuals to work closely with their healthcare team to carefully evaluate the benefits and risks of any medications or treatments they are taking. In some cases, it may be possible to find alternative treatments that are more effective or have fewer side effects. It is also important to follow the prescribed dosage and frequency of medications, and to report any changes in symptoms or side effects to a healthcare provider.

NOTES:_____

_____

Overall, medical dependency can be a complex and ongoing issue that requires careful management and monitoring to ensure that individuals are receiving the most appropriate and effective treatment for their medical condition.

## MEDITATION

Meditation is a mental exercise that involves focusing one's attention on a particular object, thought, or activity to train attention and awareness, and achieve a mentally clear and emotionally calm and stable state. It is often used for relaxation, stress reduction, and to improve overall well-being.

There are many different types of meditation practices, such as mindfulness meditation, loving-kindness meditation, and transcendental meditation. These practices can be done while sitting, standing, lying down, or even while walking or engaging in other activities. Some people may meditate in a quiet place, while others may do it while listening to music or guided meditations.

Meditation can be practiced by people of all ages and backgrounds, and it has been shown to have a number of health benefits, including reducing stress and anxiety, improving sleep, and increasing self-awareness and concentration. It is a popular form of complementary and alternative medicine, and is often recommended by healthcare providers as a way to improve overall well-being.

## MENTAL HEALTH

Mental health refers to a person's overall psychological well-being. It includes the ability to manage one's

NOTES:_____
_____

emotions, thoughts, and behaviors, as well as to cope with the challenges of daily life. Good mental health is important for overall health and well-being. It enables individuals to feel good about themselves, to form and maintain positive relationships, and to effectively cope with life's challenges.

On the other hand, poor mental health can lead to a range of problems, including difficulty with daily activities, decreased productivity, depression and increased risk of physical health problems.

Mental health issues can take many forms and can affect people of all ages, genders, and cultural backgrounds. Some common mental health conditions include depression, anxiety, bipolar disorder, and schizophrenia. Many people with mental health issues can receive treatment and lead fulfilling lives, but it is important to seek help if you are experiencing symptoms or are having difficulty managing your emotions, thoughts, or behaviors.

## METABOLISM

Metabolism refers to the chemical processes that occur within a living organism to maintain life. These processes include the conversion of food into energy, the regulation of hormones, and the maintenance of cell structure.

The body's metabolic rate, or the speed at which these processes occur, can be influenced by a variety of factors including genetics, age, sex, and overall health. A high metabolic rate can lead to weight loss, while a low metabolic rate can contribute to weight gain. Additionally, certain medical conditions such as thyroid

NOTES:_____

_____

disorders can affect metabolism and lead to changes in weight, energy levels, and overall health.

## NATURAL

The term "natural" as it pertains to ingredients in food generally refers to ingredients that are minimally processed and come from natural sources. This can include ingredients that are grown or raised, as well as ingredients that are derived from natural sources through simple processes, such as grinding or drying.

However, there is no legal definition of the term "natural" in the context of food labeling, and it is not regulated by the Food and Drug Administration (FDA) in the United States. As a result, the use of the term "natural" on food labels can be somewhat misleading and is not always a reliable indicator of the quality or healthfulness of the product. It is important to read the ingredient list and nutritional information on food labels to get a better understanding of what is in the product.

## NATURAL DIURETIC

A natural diuretic is a substance that helps to increase the production of urine in the body, which can help to flush out excess fluids and toxins. Natural diuretics can be found in a variety of foods and herbs, and they work by stimulating the kidneys to produce more urine or by inhibiting the reabsorption of water and electrolytes by the kidneys.

Some examples of natural diuretics include dandelion, asparagus, and green tea. They are often used to treat conditions such as edema (swelling due to excess fluid accumulation), high blood pressure, and kidney or liver

NOTES:_____

_____

disorders. It is important to note that natural diuretics should not be used as a replacement for medical treatment, and it is always best to consult with a healthcare provider before using any natural remedies.

There are several natural substances that can act as diuretics and increase urine production, but it is important to use caution when using these substances as diuretics. Some natural diuretics may have side effects or interact with medications, and in some cases, they may not be safe for long-term use.

Here are some examples of natural substances that may act as diuretics, but may not be healthy for long-term use:

1. Caffeine: Caffeine is a natural stimulant that is found in coffee, tea, and chocolate, and it can act as a diuretic by increasing urine production. However, caffeine can also cause side effects such as jitters, insomnia, and increased heart rate.

2. Alcohol: Alcohol can act as a diuretic by increasing urine production and can lead to dehydration. However, alcohol can also have harmful effects on the body, including liver damage and addiction.

3. Dandelion: Dandelion is a natural diuretic that is often used in herbal remedies. However, dandelion may interact with certain medications and can cause allergic reactions in some people.

4. Uva ursi: Uva ursi, also known as bearberry, is a natural diuretic that is often used in herbal remedies. However, uva ursi may interact with certain medications and can cause allergic reactions in some people.

NOTES:_____

_____

It is important to consult with a healthcare provider before using any natural diuretic, as they can interact with medications and have side effects. It is also important to drink plenty of fluids when using diuretics to prevent dehydration.

## NEGATIVE ENERGY BALANCE

A negative energy balance is a state in which the amount of energy expended by the body is greater than the amount of energy consumed. This can occur when the body is burning more calories than it is taking in through food and drink, resulting in weight loss. When it comes to weight loss a negative energy balance can have both positive and negative effects on the body.

Pros:

- **Weight loss:** When the body is in a negative energy balance, it will burn stored fat as a source of energy, leading to weight loss.

- **Improved insulin sensitivity:** A negative energy balance can also improve the body's sensitivity to insulin, which can help to prevent or manage diabetes.

- **Increased muscle mass:** When the body is in a negative energy balance, it may also increase muscle mass, as the body will burn fat for energy and spare muscle tissue.

Cons:

- **Hunger and cravings:** When the body is in a negative energy balance, it can lead to feelings of hunger and cravings for high-calorie foods.

190

- Fatigue: The body may also feel tired and weak when in a negative energy balance, as it does not have enough energy to perform daily activities.
- Nutrient deficiencies: A negative energy balance can also lead to nutrient deficiencies, as the body may not be getting enough essential vitamins and minerals from food.
- Slow metabolism: A negative energy balance can slow down the metabolism, which can make it harder to maintain weight loss over time.
- Malnutrition: A negative energy balance can lead to malnutrition over the long-term, which can cause multiple health problems.

It's important to note that a negative energy balance is not recommended for long-term weight loss or health improvement, as it can have negative effects on the body. A moderate energy deficit along with a balanced diet and exercise regimen is considered a healthier approach to weight loss.

## NET-ZERO FOOD

Net-zero food refers to the idea of balancing the nutrients that are taken in through food consumption with the nutrients that are excreted or otherwise eliminated from the body. In other words, a person's diet could be considered net-zero if the nutrients they consume through food are fully utilized by the body and there is no excess or deficiency.

The concept of net-zero food is often discussed in the context of sustainability and the environmental impact of food production. A net-zero food system would aim to minimize waste and ensure that all resources used in food production are efficiently used and not wasted.

191

In terms of the human body, a net-zero diet could potentially help to maintain optimal health and prevent nutrient deficiencies or excesses. However, it is important to note that the specific nutrients and amounts needed for optimal health can vary from person to person, depending on factors such as age, gender, weight, and level of physical activity. It is important for individuals to work with a healthcare professional or a registered dietitian to determine their individual nutrient needs and to ensure that their diet is balanced and adequately meets those needs.

## NON-GMO – NON GENETICALLY MODIFIED

Non-GMO, or non-genetically modified organisms, refers to products that do not contain genetically modified ingredients or materials derived from genetically modified organisms. Genetically modified organisms (GMOs) are plants or animals that have had their DNA altered or modified in some way through genetic engineering. This is typically done to give the organism a desired trait or characteristic, such as resistance to pests or increased crop yield.

There is ongoing debate about the safety and potential risks of genetically modified organisms, with some people expressing concerns about their impact on the environment and human health. As a result, some people choose to consume non-GMO products as a way to avoid genetically modified ingredients. Non-GMO products can be found in a variety of categories, including food, personal care products, and household items.

I personally try to avoid genetically modified foods, so I look for "Non-GMO" on most of the packaged foods I purchase, but it also pertains to fresh produce, which can also be genetically modified, which is why I

NOTES:_____
_____

purchased organic produce. To be called organic, it must not be genetically modified.

## NUTRITION

Nutrition refers to the intake of nutrients that are necessary for the proper functioning of the human body. These nutrients include carbohydrates, proteins, fats, vitamins, minerals, and water. Nutrition is important for maintaining good health and for the prevention of various diseases. Adequate nutrition helps to ensure that the body has the energy it needs to perform its daily functions, such as physical activity, growth, and repair. It also helps to support the immune system, which helps to protect the body from infection and illness. Poor nutrition can lead to a variety of health problems, including malnutrition, deficiencies, and chronic diseases such as obesity, type 2 diabetes, and heart disease.

There are many important nutrients that the human body needs to function properly. Some examples include:

1. Protein: an essential nutrient that is necessary for the growth, repair, and maintenance of tissues in the body. It is also important for the production of hormones, enzymes, and other molecules that play important roles in the body.

2. Carbohydrates: a type of nutrient that is important for providing energy to the body, particularly for the brain and muscles. There are different types of carbohydrates, including simple sugars and complex carbohydrates, which are found in a variety of foods such as fruits, vegetables, grains, and legumes.

193

NOTES:_____

_____

3. Fats: a type of nutrient that is important for providing energy to the body and helping to absorb and transport certain vitamins and minerals. Fats also play a role in maintaining healthy skin and hair, and they are a source of essential fatty acids, which are necessary for proper brain function and overall health.

4. Vitamins: micronutrients that are essential for the proper functioning of the body. There are many different types of vitamins, including vitamins A, B, C, D, E, and K, which are found in a variety of foods such as fruits, vegetables, and grains.

5. Minerals: micronutrients that are essential for maintaining the proper balance of electrolytes in the body and for supporting various functions such as bone health, nerve function, and muscle function. Examples of minerals include calcium, iron, sodium, and potassium.

6. Water: an essential nutrient that is necessary for the proper functioning of all body systems. Water helps to regulate body temperature, transport nutrients and oxygen to cells, and flush out waste products. It is important to drink plenty of water throughout the day to stay hydrated.

OBESITY

According to data from the Centers for Disease Control and Prevention (CDC), about 42.4% of adults in the United States are obese. Obesity is defined as having a body mass index (BMI) of 30 or higher.

In addition, the CDC reports that about 13.7% of adults in the United States have extreme obesity, defined as a BMI of 40 or higher. Obesity is a serious health issue

NOTES:_____
_____

because it is associated with an increased risk of a number of serious health conditions, including heart disease, stroke, type 2 diabetes, and some types of cancer.

Obesity is also a significant contributor to health care costs in the United States. In 2018, the estimated annual medical cost of obesity was $147 billion.

It's important to note that these statistics apply to adults, and the prevalence of obesity and extreme obesity may be different among children and teenagers. The CDC also reports that about 18.5% of children and adolescents in the United States are obese.

Being overweight, defined as having a body mass index (BMI) of 25 or above, is associated with a number of serious health issues. Here are some of the most significant health problems linked to being overweight:

1. Cardiovascular disease: Overweight individuals are at an increased risk of developing heart disease, high blood pressure, and stroke. This is due to the fact that excess weight puts extra strain on the heart and blood vessels, leading to an increased risk of plaque buildup in the arteries and blood clots.

2. Diabetes: Overweight individuals are at an increased risk of developing type 2 diabetes, which occurs when the body becomes resistant to insulin or doesn't produce enough of it. Insulin is a hormone that helps regulate blood sugar levels, and high blood sugar levels can lead to serious health problems, including nerve damage, kidney damage, and vision loss.

3. Cancer: Being overweight has been linked to an increased risk of developing certain types of cancer, including breast, colon, and endometrial cancer.

195

NOTES:_____

_____

4. Osteoarthritis: Being overweight can increase the risk of developing osteoarthritis, a degenerative joint disease that causes pain and stiffness in the joints. The extra weight puts added stress on the joints, which can lead to wear and tear over time.

5. Sleep apnea: Overweight individuals are more likely to develop sleep apnea, a sleep disorder characterized by pauses in breathing during sleep. Sleep apnea can lead to fatigue, irritability, and other health problems.

6. Gallstones: Excess weight can increase the risk of developing gallstones, which are small, hard stones that form in the gallbladder. Gallstones can cause abdominal pain and discomfort and may require medical treatment.

In addition to these health issues, being overweight can also lead to social and psychological problems, such as discrimination, low self-esteem, and depression. It is important for individuals who are overweight to take steps to achieve and maintain a healthy weight in order to reduce their risk of these serious health problems. This may involve lifestyle changes, such as eating a healthy diet and getting regular physical activity, as well as seeking the guidance of a healthcare professional.


## OMEGA-3 FATTY ACIDS

Omega-3 fatty acids are a type of polyunsaturated fat that are important for maintaining good health. They are called "omega-3s" because they are the third type of fat in the series of fatty acids that begin with omega-3. Omega-3s are found in a variety of foods, including fatty fish, nuts, and seeds. They are known to have anti-inflammatory properties and have been shown to have a number of health benefits, including reducing the risk of

196

NOTES:_____

heart disease and stroke, improving cognitive function, and reducing the risk of certain types of cancer. They are also important for maintaining healthy skin and hair, and for supporting the development and function of the brain, eyes, and immune system.

## ORGANIC FOOD

Organic refers to the way agricultural products are grown and processed. Organic farming methods rely on natural processes, such as crop rotation and composting, to enhance soil fertility and control pests and diseases. Organic foods are produced without the use of synthetic pesticides, fertilizers, genetically modified organisms (GMOs), irradiation, or other artificial additives or processing aids. Organic products also must be produced using sustainable farming practices that protect the environment and animal welfare.

There are several potential benefits to eating organic foods. Here are a few:

1. Fewer pesticides: Organic farming practices generally involve using fewer pesticides and fertilizers, which can be beneficial for both human health and the environment.

2. More nutrients: Some studies have found that organic produce may contain higher levels of certain nutrients, such as vitamin C and antioxidants, compared to conventionally grown produce.

3. Better flavor: Many people believe that organic foods taste better than conventionally grown foods. This could be because organic farming practices often involve using methods that

197

NOTES:_____

_____

prioritize the quality of the soil, which can lead to more flavorful produce.

4. No genetically modified organisms (GMOs): Organic foods are not allowed to be produced using genetically modified organisms (GMOs). Some people choose to eat organic foods to avoid consuming GMOs.

5. Supporting small farmers and sustainability: Organic farming is often associated with small, local farms that prioritize sustainability and humane treatment of animals. By choosing organic foods, you may be supporting these types of farms and their values.

It's worth noting that while organic foods may offer some potential benefits, there is still ongoing debate about whether they are nutritionally superior to conventionally grown foods. It's also important to keep in mind that organic foods can be more expensive than conventionally grown foods, so it may not be feasible for everyone to eat a completely organic diet.

## PALEO DIET

The paleo diet, also known as the "caveman diet" or the "stone age diet," is a dietary plan based on the idea that modern humans should eat like their prehistoric ancestors. This means that the diet consists mainly of whole, unprocessed foods such as fruits, vegetables, meats, and nuts, and excludes foods that were not available or were not commonly consumed during the Paleolithic era, such as dairy products, grains, legumes, and processed foods.

Proponents of the paleo diet argue that it can improve health and reduce the risk of chronic diseases by

NOTES:_____

_____

eliminating certain types of foods that may be harmful or inflammatory for some people. However, the scientific evidence for the effectiveness of the paleo diet is mixed, and it may not be suitable for everyone. It is important to consult with a healthcare provider or a registered dietitian before starting any new diet.


## PESCATARIAN

A pescatarian is a person who abstains from eating meat and poultry, but includes fish and other seafood in their diet. Pescatarians may also include other animal products such as eggs and dairy in their diet. This type of dietary choice may be motivated by a variety of factors, including health, environmental concerns, or ethical concerns about animal welfare.

 Pescatararianism can be seen as a type of semi-vegetarianism, as it involves abstaining from some types of animal protein while still consuming others.

## pH – POTENTIAL OF HYDROGEN

pH is a measure of hydrogen ion concentration, a measure of the acidity or alkalinity of a solution. The pH scale ranges from 0 to 14.

A solution with a pH of 7 is considered neutral, meaning that it has equal concentrations of H+ and OH- ions. Solutions with a pH less than 7 are considered acidic, while those with a pH greater than 7 are considered alkaline.

The pH scale is logarithmic, meaning that each increment on the scale represents a tenfold difference in acidity or alkalinity. For example, a solution with a pH of 5 is ten times more acidic than a solution with a pH of 6,

199

and a solution with a pH of 9 is ten times more alkaline than a solution with a pH of 8.

The pH of a solution can be measured using a pH meter or pH strips. These tools use a probe or indicator to measure the concentration of H+ ions in the solution. The pH can also be calculated using the concentration of hydrogen ions in a solution using the equation: $pH = -\log[H+]$.

The pH of a solution can be affected by the presence of acids or bases. An acid is a substance that donates H+ ions to a solution, while a base is a substance that accepts H+ ions. The pH of a solution can also be affected by the concentration of dissolved ions, the temperature, and the presence of buffers.

Buffers are substances that can absorb excess H+ ions or OH- ions in a solution, helping to maintain a relatively constant pH. They are important in many biological systems, where the pH must be maintained within a narrow range for enzymes and other proteins to function properly.


## PHYSICAL ACTIVITY

Physical activity and staying fit are important for a number of reasons.

First and foremost, regular physical activity is essential for maintaining good physical health. It helps to strengthen the muscles, bones, and joints, improve cardiovascular health, and reduce the risk of developing chronic conditions such as obesity, heart disease, and type 2 diabetes. It can also help to reduce the risk of certain cancers, such as breast and colon cancer.

In addition to the physical benefits, regular physical activity can also have a positive impact on mental

NOTES:_____
_____

health. Exercise can help to reduce stress, improve mood, and increase self-esteem. It can also improve sleep quality and help to alleviate anxiety and depression.

Staying fit can also improve overall quality of life. It can increase energy levels, improve mobility, and make daily activities such as climbing stairs or carrying groceries easier.

Overall, the importance of physical activity and staying fit cannot be overstated. It is essential for both physical and mental well-being, and has the potential to greatly improve quality of life.

Here are just a few of the many benefits of staying active and fit:

1. Improved cardiovascular health: Regular physical activity can help improve your cardiovascular health by strengthening your heart and reducing your risk of heart disease.

2. Stronger muscles and bones: Exercise can help strengthen your muscles and bones, reducing your risk of osteoporosis and falls.

3. Weight management: Physical activity can help you maintain a healthy weight or lose weight if needed.

4. Improved mental health: Regular exercise has been shown to improve mood and reduce stress, anxiety, and depression.

5. Better sleep: Exercise can help improve sleep quality and quantity.

6. Increased energy: Being active can help boost your energy levels and increase your stamina.

7. Improved cognitive function: Exercise has been shown to improve brain function, including

201

memory, concentration, and decision-making skills.

8. Increased flexibility: Staying active can help improve your flexibility and range of motion.

9. Enhanced immune function: Exercise has been shown to boost the immune system and help reduce the risk of illness.

10. Improved self-esteem: Being physically active and fit can improve self-esteem and body image.

## PREBIOTICS

Prebiotics are non-digestible dietary fibers that stimulate the growth and activity of beneficial bacteria in the gut. They are found in a variety of foods, including vegetables, fruits, whole grains, and legumes. Prebiotics are thought to have a number of health benefits, including supporting the immune system, improving digestion, and possibly even helping to prevent certain diseases. It is important to consume a varied diet that includes a variety of prebiotics in order to support the growth of a diverse range of beneficial bacteria in the gut.

## PRESCRIPTION MEDICATION

Prescription medications can have potential risks and side effects, just like any other type of medication. It is important to be aware of these risks and to discuss them with your healthcare provider before starting a new prescription.

Some common potential risks and side effects of prescription medications include:

202

1. Allergic reactions: Some people may have an allergic reaction to a medication, which can cause symptoms such as rash, hives, difficulty breathing, and swelling of the face, lips, tongue, or throat.

2. Interactions with other medications: Certain medications can interact with each other and cause unintended side effects. It is important to inform your healthcare provider about all the medications you are taking, including over-the-counter drugs, herbs, and supplements, to help avoid potential interactions.

3. Dosage issues: Taking too much of a medication or taking it too frequently can lead to overdose, which can cause serious side effects and even death. On the other hand, not taking a medication as prescribed or skipping doses can lead to reduced effectiveness or even harm. It is important to follow your healthcare provider's instructions for taking your medication.

4. Side effects: Every medication has the potential to cause side effects, which can range from mild to severe. Common side effects may include nausea, dizziness, headache, and drowsiness. More serious side effects may include changes in blood pressure, liver damage, and kidney damage. It is important to report any side effects to your healthcare provider.

It is important to remember that although prescription medications can have risks and side effects, they can also be very effective at treating various health conditions. It is important to work with your healthcare provider to determine the best treatment plan for you, which may include prescription medications.

NOTES:_____

_____

# PRESERVATIVES

Preservatives are substances that are added to processed food to help extend its shelf life by preventing spoilage and deterioration. There are several types of preservatives that are used in food processing, including antimicrobial agents, antioxidants, and pH control agents.

Antimicrobial agents are used to prevent the growth of microorganisms, such as bacteria, fungi, and yeasts, which can cause food to spoil or become unsafe to eat. Examples of antimicrobial agents that are commonly used as food preservatives include sodium benzoate, potassium sorbate, and propionic acid.

Antioxidants are used to prevent the oxidation of food, which can lead to the loss of flavor, color, and nutritional value. Examples of antioxidants that are commonly used as food preservatives include vitamin E (tocopherol), ascorbic acid (vitamin C), and BHA (butylated hydroxyanisole).

pH control agents are used to adjust the acidity or basicity of a food product, which can help to preserve its quality and stability. Examples of pH control agents that are commonly used as food preservatives include citric acid and sodium citrate.

It's important to note that while preservatives can help to extend the shelf life of processed food, they may also have potential health risks if consumed in large amounts. Therefore, it is important to read food labels carefully and choose processed foods that are made with minimal amounts of preservatives.

Preservatives are added to food and other products to help prevent spoilage and extend shelf life. Some preservatives have been linked to potential health

NOTES:_____

concerns, although the extent of the risks varies depending on the specific preservative and the amount consumed. Here are some potential hazards of consuming preservatives:

1. Allergic reactions: Some people may have an allergic reaction to certain preservatives, such as sodium benzoate or potassium bisulfite. Symptoms of an allergic reaction may include skin rash, hives, itching, difficulty breathing, and swelling of the face, lips, tongue, or throat.

2. Toxic effects: Some preservatives, such as sodium benzoate and propylene glycol, have been linked to toxic effects when consumed in large amounts. These effects may include organ damage and neurological problems.

3. Cancer risk: Some studies have suggested that certain preservatives, such as sodium benzoate and nitrites, may increase the risk of cancer when consumed in large amounts over a long period of time. However, the evidence for these potential risks is not conclusive, and more research is needed to fully understand the potential health effects of these preservatives.

It's important to note that preservatives are added to food and other products in small amounts and are generally considered safe when consumed at normal levels. However, if you are concerned about the potential risks of consuming preservatives, you may want to consider choosing foods and products that are free of preservatives or that contain natural preservatives, such as vinegar or lemon juice.

NOTES:_____

## PROBIOTICS

Probiotics are living microorganisms, usually bacteria, that are similar to the beneficial microorganisms found in the human gut. They are sometimes called "good" or "helpful" bacteria because they help keep the gut healthy. Probiotics are found in some foods, such as yogurt and sauerkraut, and they are also available as dietary supplements.

Probiotics are thought to have a number of health benefits, including improving digestion and helping to maintain the balance of microorganisms in the gut. Some research has also suggested that probiotics may help to reduce the risk of certain types of infections and improve immune function. However, more research is needed to fully understand the potential benefits of probiotics.

It's important to note that probiotics are not a replacement for a healthy diet and lifestyle. If you are considering taking probiotics, it's a good idea to talk to your healthcare provider to determine if they are appropriate for you and to discuss the proper dosage.

Probiotics are live microorganisms that are similar to the beneficial microorganisms found in the human gut. They are often called "good" or "helpful" bacteria because they can help keep the gut healthy. Probiotics are found in a variety of foods, including:

1. Yogurt: Many brands of yogurt contain live and active cultures of probiotics.
2. Kefir: This fermented milk drink is made with kefir grains, which contain a variety of beneficial microorganisms.

NOTES:_____

_____

3. Sauerkraut: This fermented cabbage dish is a good source of probiotics, as it is made with lactic acid bacteria.

4. Kimchi: This spicy fermented cabbage dish is a traditional Korean food that is rich in probiotics.

5. Miso: This fermented soybean paste is a staple in Japanese cuisine and is a good source of probiotics.

6. Pickles: Some pickles are made through the process of fermentation, which can result in the growth of probiotics.

7. Tempeh: This fermented soybean product is a staple in Indonesian cuisine and is a good source of probiotics.

8. Kombucha: This fermented tea drink is made with a symbiotic culture of bacteria and yeast (SCOBY) and is a good source of probiotics.

It's worth noting that not all types of fermented foods contain probiotics, as the specific microorganisms present can vary. Some products, such as yogurt and kefir, are specifically formulated to contain specific strains of probiotics.

## PROCESSED FOOD

Processed foods are foods that have undergone a series of steps to transform them from their raw or natural state into something that is ready for consumption. These steps may include washing, chopping, freezing, canning, drying, grinding, and mixing, among others. Processed foods may also be treated with preservatives, flavorings, or other additives to improve their shelf life, taste, or appearance.

NOTES:_____

_____

Examples of processed foods include frozen dinners, canned soups, snack foods, and packaged baked goods. Some processed foods can be a convenient and nutritious part of a healthy diet, but others may be high in added sugars, salt, or unhealthy fats, and should be consumed in moderation.

Processed foods are foods that have been altered from their natural state for convenience, preservation, or other purposes. These foods often contain added sugars, unhealthy fats, and other additives, and may lack important nutrients found in whole, unprocessed foods.

Eating too much processed food can increase the risk of several health problems.

1. Weight gain: Processed foods are often high in calories, sugar, and unhealthy fats, which can contribute to weight gain and obesity.

2. Heart disease: Processed foods may contain high levels of sodium, which can increase blood pressure and the risk of heart disease. They may also contain unhealthy fats, such as trans fats and saturated fats, which can increase cholesterol levels and the risk of heart disease.

3. Diabetes: Processed foods may contain high levels of added sugars, which can increase the risk of type 2 diabetes.

4. Cancer: Some studies have suggested that a diet high in processed foods may increase the risk of certain types of cancer, such as colon, breast, and prostate cancer.

5. Nutrient deficiencies: Processed foods may be lacking in important nutrients, such as fiber, vitamins, and minerals, which are essential for

208

NOTES:_____
_____

optimal health. A diet high in processed foods may lead to nutrient deficiencies over time.

It is important to remember that it is not necessary to completely eliminate processed foods from the diet, but rather to limit their intake and choose healthier options when possible. Instead of relying on processed foods as the main source of nutrition, it is important to incorporate a variety of whole, unprocessed foods into the diet, including fruits, vegetables, whole grains, and lean proteins.

## PROTEIN

Protein is an essential nutrient that plays many important roles in the human body. It is a macronutrient, meaning that the body needs relatively large amounts of it to function properly.

Proteins are made up of long chains of amino acids, which are small molecules that can be linked together in various combinations to form different types of proteins. There are 20 different amino acids that the body uses to build proteins, and the body can synthesize most of them. However, there are nine amino acids that the body cannot synthesize and must obtain through the diet, known as the essential amino acids.

Protein is important for building and repairing tissues, producing enzymes and hormones, and transporting molecules throughout the body. It is also an important source of energy, particularly during times of calorie restriction or increased physical activity.

Proteins are found in a variety of foods, including meat, poultry, fish, beans, nuts, and dairy products. It is important to consume a variety of protein-rich foods to ensure that the body gets all of the essential amino acids it needs.

209

There are nine essential amino acids that the human body cannot synthesize on its own and must obtain through diet. These are:

1. Histidine
2. Isoleucine
3. Leucine
4. Lysine
5. Methionine
6. Phenylalanine
7. Threonine
8. Tryptophan
9. Valine

Essential amino acids are important for many functions in the body, including building and repairing tissues, producing enzymes and hormones, and supporting immune system function. They are necessary for good health and proper growth and development.

## QUICK FIX

A quick fix in relation to diet refers to a short-term solution or method that is intended to produce rapid or immediate results, usually without addressing the underlying cause of a problem. Quick fixes in dieting often involve drastic or extreme measures such as crash diets, fasting, or taking weight loss supplements, and they are often marketed as an easy way to lose weight or improve health. While they may produce some initial results, they are often not sustainable in the long term and may have negative side effects, such as nutrient deficiencies or negative impacts on mental health. Instead of seeking quick fixes, it is generally more effective to adopt healthy, balanced eating habits

210

and an active lifestyle in order to achieve and maintain a healthy weight and overall health.

## RECOVERY

In the context of the human body, recovery refers to the process of repairing and rebuilding tissues and systems that have been damaged or weakened. This can involve rest, physical therapy, and other forms of treatment and rehabilitation. Recovery is an important aspect of maintaining overall health and well-being, as it helps to ensure that the body is able to function properly and perform at its best. It is a key component of many medical and healthcare practices, and is often focused on improving physical, mental, and emotional health and well-being.

## REFINED SUGAR

Refined sugar is a type of sugar that has undergone a process of refining in order to remove impurities and other substances. This process typically involves grinding the sugar cane or sugar beet into a fine powder and then treating it with chemicals to remove any impurities, such as plant debris or molasses. The resulting product is a pure, white, granulated sugar that is commonly used in cooking and baking. Refined sugar is often used as a sweetener in a variety of food and beverage products, including cereals, baked goods, and sodas. It is also used as a preservative and flavor enhancer in many processed foods. While refined sugar is a popular sweetener, it has been linked to a number of negative health effects, including tooth decay and an increased risk of obesity and other chronic diseases.

Consuming large amounts of refined sugar has been linked to a number of negative health effects. Some of

NOTES:_____

_____

the potential health hazards of consuming too much refined sugar include:

1.  Weight gain: Refined sugar is high in calories and can contribute to weight gain when consumed in excess.

2.  Dental cavities: The bacteria in the mouth can convert refined sugar into acid, which can weaken tooth enamel and lead to cavities.

3.  Insulin resistance: Consuming too much refined sugar can lead to insulin resistance, which can increase the risk of developing type 2 diabetes.

4.  Heart disease: Some studies have suggested that a high intake of refined sugars may increase the risk of heart disease.

5.  Inflammation: Consuming large amounts of refined sugar has been linked to increased inflammation in the body, which has been associated with a number of chronic diseases.

6.  Poor nutrition: Consuming a diet high in refined sugars may displace more nutritious foods, leading to a lack of important nutrients and vitamins.

It's important to note that these health hazards are associated with consuming large amounts of refined sugar, rather than small amounts consumed occasionally as part of a balanced diet. It's generally recommended to limit the intake of added sugars, including refined sugar, in order to maintain good health.


## SELF-CARE

Self-care refers to the actions that individuals take to maintain and improve their physical, mental, and

NOTES:_____

_____

emotional health. It involves taking care of one's body, mind, and spirit through activities that nourish and support overall well-being. This can include activities such as getting enough sleep, eating a healthy diet, exercising regularly, managing stress, and engaging in activities that bring joy and relaxation. Self-care is an important part of maintaining overall health and well-being, and it can help individuals feel more energized, focused, and resilient. It can also help an individual better cope with stress, illness, and other challenges that may arise in their lives.

## SODA

Soda has changed over the years and most have become filled with chemicals, artificial flavors and are loaded with refined sugar. It is generally recommended to mainly consume water as a part of a healthy diet. No matter what your weight loss goals may be, eliminating soda from your diet is strongly advised. In fact, if you are going to do anything to improve your health, cutting out soda should be at the top of your list!

I created a little rhyme to help people remember the potential hazards of drinking carbonated beverages and I hope you'll remember it and take the message to heart.

If it's got bubbles, it leads to troubles!

Drinking soda can have a number of negative effects on your health. Here are the top 10 health issues that are linked with drinking soda:

1. Weight gain: Soda is high in calories, which can contribute to weight gain and obesity.

2. Tooth decay: The high sugar content in soda can cause tooth decay and erosion of the enamel on your teeth.

213

NOTES:_____

_____

3. Type 2 diabetes: Drinking soda regularly has been linked to an increased risk of developing type 2 diabetes.

4. Heart disease: The high levels of sugar and caffeine in soda can increase the risk of heart disease.

5. Kidney problems: Consuming too much soda has been linked to an increased risk of developing kidney problems, such as kidney stones and kidney disease.

6. Osteoporosis: The high levels of phosphoric acid in soda can interfere with the body's ability to absorb calcium, which can lead to osteoporosis.

7. High blood pressure: The caffeine in soda can increase blood pressure, which can increase the risk of heart attack and stroke.

8. Metabolic syndrome: Drinking soda has been linked to an increased risk of developing metabolic syndrome, a group of conditions that increase the risk of heart disease, stroke, and diabetes.

9. Liver problems: Consuming too much soda has been linked to an increased risk of developing non-alcoholic fatty liver disease.

10. Gout: The high levels of purines in soda can increase the risk of developing gout, a form of arthritis that causes inflammation and pain in the joints.

There are many compelling reasons to avoid drinking soda. It is high in sugar, can contribute to tooth decay, has little nutritional value, contains caffeine, and can have negative environmental impacts. Choosing water as your main beverage of choice can help support overall health and well-being.

NOTES:_____

_____

## SODIUM / SALT

Sodium, also referred to as salt, is in almost every premade or processed food. Salt has been very important to people for thousands of years and is actually one of the essential minerals needed for health. However, eating too much salt can have negative effects on your health. Consuming high levels of salt can lead to an increased risk of developing high blood pressure, also known as hypertension. High blood pressure is a major risk factor for cardiovascular diseases such as heart attacks and stroke.

When you eat a lot of salt, your body holds onto extra water to dilute the sodium. This can cause your blood volume to increase, which puts extra strain on your blood vessels and heart. Over time, this can lead to high blood pressure and other health problems.

In addition to increasing the risk of cardiovascular disease, consuming too much salt can also contribute to other health problems. It can lead to fluid retention, which can cause swelling in the hands, feet, and ankles. It can also worsen some digestive disorders and contribute to the development of kidney stones.

The recommended daily intake of salt is less than 2,300 milligrams per day for adults. However, the average American consumes closer to 3,400 milligrams of salt per day, which is well above the recommended amount. To reduce your salt intake, try to limit your intake of processed and packaged foods, which are often high in sodium. Instead, opt for fresh, whole foods and consider using herbs and spices to add flavor to your meals.

Eating too much salt can lead to several health problems, including:

1. High blood pressure: Salt can cause your body to retain fluid, which can increase blood pressure.

215

NOTES:_____

_____

High blood pressure is a major risk factor for heart disease and stroke.

2. Kidney damage: Your kidneys are responsible for removing excess salt from your body. If you eat too much salt, your kidneys may not be able to keep up, which can lead to kidney damage over time.

3. Osteoporosis: High salt intake can interfere with the balance of calcium in your body, which can lead to osteoporosis, a condition that causes your bones to become weak and brittle.

4. Stomach cancer: Some studies have suggested that a high salt intake may increase the risk of stomach cancer.

5. Heart disease: High salt intake has been linked to an increased risk of heart disease, as it can lead to high blood pressure and other factors that contribute to heart disease.

It's important to consume salt in moderation and to choose foods that are low in salt when possible. The American Heart Association recommends that adults consume no more than 2,300 milligrams of sodium per day, and that those with high blood pressure, diabetes, or chronic kidney disease aim for no more than 1,500 milligrams per day.


## STRESS

Stress is a normal part of life and can be caused by a variety of factors, including work, relationships, and personal problems. When we experience stress, our bodies respond by releasing stress hormones, such as adrenaline and cortisol, which can affect our physical and mental well-being.

NOTES:_____

_____

It's important to note that everyone responds to stress differently, and the effects of stress can vary depending on the severity and duration of the stress. Some people may be more resilient to stress and able to cope with it more effectively, while others may be more vulnerable and experience more negative effects.

It's important to manage stress in order to maintain good physical and mental health. Some ways to manage stress include practicing relaxation techniques such as deep breathing or meditation, exercising regularly, and getting enough sleep. It's also important to eat a healthy diet, stay hydrated, and connect with others for support. If you're experiencing significant stress that is affecting your daily life, it may be helpful to seek support from a mental health professional.

Stress can affect your health in a number of ways. Here are some examples of how stress can impact your physical and mental health:

1. Physical symptoms: Stress can cause physical symptoms such as headache, muscle tension, stomach upset, and fatigue.

2. Mental health problems: Stress can contribute to the development of mental health problems such as anxiety and depression.

3. Heart disease: Chronic stress has been linked to an increased risk of heart disease.

4. Type 2 diabetes: Stress can cause blood sugar levels to rise, which can increase the risk of developing type 2 diabetes.

5. Digestive problems: Stress can disrupt the digestive process, leading to issues such as stomach pain, bloating, and diarrhea.

6. Sleep problems: Stress can interfere with sleep, causing difficulty falling asleep or staying asleep.

217

7. Weakened immune system: Stress can weaken the immune system, making you more susceptible to illness.

8. Weight gain: Stress can cause changes in appetite and metabolism, leading to weight gain.

There are a number of ways to cope with stress and reduce its negative effects on our bodies and minds. Some strategies for managing stress include:

1. Identifying the sources of stress: Understanding what is causing your stress can help you take steps to address the problem or find ways to cope with it.

2. Practicing relaxation techniques: Deep breathing, meditation, and progressive muscle relaxation are all effective ways to relax and calm the mind and body.

3. Exercising regularly: Physical activity can help reduce stress by releasing endorphins and improving overall physical and mental health.

4. Getting enough sleep: Adequate sleep can help you cope with stress and maintain good physical and mental health.

5. Eating a healthy diet: A balanced diet can help you maintain energy and cope with stress more effectively.

6. Seeking support: Talking to friends, family, or a therapist can be a helpful way to cope with stress and gain perspective on problems.

7. Setting boundaries: Learning to say no and setting limits can help you manage your time and energy, reducing the risk of becoming overwhelmed by stress.

NOTES:_____

_____

8. Finding ways to manage time effectively: Prioritizing tasks and setting achievable goals can help you feel more in control and reduce stress.

9. Seeking professional help: If you are unable to cope with stress on your own, it may be helpful to seek the support of a mental health professional, such as a therapist or counselor.

By adopting a combination of these stress-management strategies, you can learn to effectively cope with stress and improve your overall well-being.

## SUGAR ALCOHOL

Sugar alcohols are a type of low-calorie sweetener that are commonly used in processed foods as a sugar substitute. They are found naturally in some fruits and vegetables and can also be produced artificially through chemical processes. Sugar alcohols are chemically similar to both sugars and alcohols, but they do not contain ethanol (the type of alcohol found in alcoholic beverages).

Sugar alcohols are not as sweet as regular sugar, and they are absorbed more slowly by the body, which means they can provide a lower-calorie alternative to sugar in food and drink products. They are often used in products such as low-calorie and sugar-free candies, gum, baked goods, and other processed foods.

Some common types of sugar alcohols include xylitol, erythritol, lactitol, and maltitol. These sweeteners are generally considered safe for consumption, but they can have a laxative effect in some people if consumed in large amounts. It is important to read the ingredient labels on food products to determine whether they

NOTES:_____

_____

contain sugar alcohols and to be aware of the potential effects on your body.

## SUGAR-FREE

Sugar-free is a term used to describe food and drinks that do not contain any added sugar. Sugar-free products may contain artificial sweeteners or other sugar substitutes in place of sugar to provide a sweet taste. The term "sugar-free" can be used to describe a wide range of products, including beverages, desserts, condiments, and more.

Some people choose to consume sugar-free products as a way to reduce their intake of added sugars, which are linked to a variety of health issues, including obesity, type 2 diabetes, and tooth decay. However, it is important to note that sugar-free products may still contain calories and may not necessarily be healthier than their regular counterparts.

It's important to note that just because a food is sugar-free does not necessarily mean that it is bad for the body. In fact, many sugar-free foods can be a healthy and nutritious choice. However, it is still important to read labels and ingredient lists carefully, as some sugar-free foods may still contain other potentially harmful ingredients.

Here are a few examples of sugar-free foods that may be potentially harmful if consumed in excess:

1.  Sugar-free gums and mints: These products often contain sugar substitutes such as xylitol or aspartame, which can have negative effects on the body when consumed in large amounts.

2.  Sugar-free baked goods: These products may contain sugar substitutes such as maltitol, which

NOTES:_____

_____

can have a laxative effect when consumed in large amounts.

3. Sugar-free drinks: Some sugar-free drinks, such as diet sodas, contain artificial sweeteners like aspartame, which have been linked to a variety of health issues when consumed in excess.

It's important to remember that all foods, including sugar-free ones, should be consumed in moderation as part of a balanced diet. It is also a good idea to speak with a healthcare professional if you have any concerns about the safety of a particular food or ingredient.

## SUPERFOOD

A superfood is a type of food that is considered to be particularly nutritious and beneficial for health. These foods are typically high in antioxidants, vitamins, minerals, and other nutrients that are essential for maintaining good health.

Some examples of superfoods include berries, leafy green vegetables, nuts, seeds, and whole grains. Many people believe that including superfoods in their diet can help to prevent or mitigate various health problems, such as heart disease, diabetes, and cancer. However, it is important to note that no single food can provide all of the nutrients that the body needs, and a varied and balanced diet is the key to good health.

Superfoods are foods that are nutrient-rich and provide numerous health benefits. Some examples of superfoods include:

1. Blueberries: These small, sweet fruits are high in antioxidants, which may help protect against cell damage and reduce the risk of certain diseases.

221

2. Salmon: This type of fish is high in omega-3 fatty acids, which are important for brain health and may help reduce the risk of heart disease.

3. Spinach: This leafy green is high in vitamins and minerals, including vitamin K, vitamin A, and folate. It also contains antioxidants that may help protect against cancer and other diseases.

4. Avocado: This fruit is high in healthy fats, which may help improve cholesterol levels and reduce the risk of heart disease. It is also a good source of fiber, potassium, and vitamins E and C.

5. Nuts: Nuts, such as almonds, walnuts, and pistachios, are high in healthy fats, protein, and fiber. They may help improve cholesterol levels and reduce the risk of heart disease.

6. Chia seeds: These tiny seeds are high in fiber, protein, and omega-3 fatty acids. They may help improve digestion, reduce the risk of heart disease, and lower cholesterol levels.

7. Dark chocolate: This type of chocolate is high in antioxidants, which may help protect against cell damage and reduce the risk of certain diseases. It is also a good source of iron, magnesium, and zinc.

8. Turmeric: This spice is high in curcumin, which has anti-inflammatory properties and may help reduce the risk of certain diseases.

9. Green tea: This tea is high in antioxidants, which may help protect against cell damage and reduce the risk of certain diseases. It is also a good source of catechins, which may have a variety of health benefits.

10. Goji berries: These small, red berries are high in antioxidants and may have a variety of health

NOTES:_____

_____

benefits, including improving immune function and reducing the risk of certain diseases.

## SUPPLEMENTS

Supplements are substances that are usually taken orally and are intended to supplement the diet. They are usually in the form of pills, capsules, powders, or liquids, and are intended to provide nutrients that may not be consumed in sufficient quantities in a person's diet. Some common types of supplements include vitamins, minerals, amino acids, and herbs.

Supplements may be used to treat a deficiency or imbalance in the body, to support certain body functions, or to support overall health and wellness. It is important to note that supplements are not intended to replace a balanced diet, and it is always best to try to obtain nutrients from natural sources whenever possible.

It is also important to talk to a healthcare professional before starting any supplement regimen, as some supplements can interact with medications or have potential side effects.

## TOXINS

Toxins are substances that are harmful or poisonous to the human body. They can be found in a variety of sources, including the environment, certain foods and beverages, and certain medications. Toxins can enter the body through ingestion, inhalation, or skin contact, and they can have a variety of negative effects on the body, ranging from mild symptoms such as dizziness

223

NOTES:_____

_____

and nausea to more serious effects such as organ damage or even death.

Some common toxins include heavy metals, pesticides, and chemicals found in tobacco smoke and industrial pollutants. It is important to be aware of the potential sources of toxins and to take steps to reduce exposure to them in order to maintain good health.

## VEGAN

Being vegan is a lifestyle and dietary choice that involves abstaining from using animal products for food, clothing, and other purposes. This includes avoiding meat, dairy, eggs, and honey, as well as products that are made from animal by-products such as leather, wool, and silk.

There are many reasons why someone might choose to follow a vegan lifestyle. Some people do it for ethical reasons, as they believe that it is wrong to exploit and harm animals for human benefit. Others may adopt a vegan lifestyle for health reasons, as a vegan diet can be high in nutrients and low in saturated fat and cholesterol. Some people also choose veganism as a way to reduce their environmental impact, as animal agriculture can be a major contributor to greenhouse gas emissions and deforestation.

While veganism can have many benefits, it is important to ensure that you are meeting all of your nutritional needs when following this type of diet. This may require careful planning and the use of fortified foods or supplements to ensure that you are getting enough protein, vitamins, and minerals. It is also important to be mindful of any food allergies or sensitivities that you may have and to choose appropriate plant-based alternatives.

224

One challenge that vegans may face is finding suitable options when eating out or traveling. Many restaurants and cafes now offer vegan options, but it may be necessary to make special requests or do research in advance to find places that cater to vegan diets. It is also a good idea to carry some vegan snacks with you in case you are unable to find suitable options while on the go.

In conclusion, being vegan is a personal choice that can have a variety of motivations and benefits. While it may require some extra planning and consideration, it is possible to follow a healthy and satisfying vegan lifestyle with the right knowledge and resources.

My family and I was vegan for almost two years. During this time we ate a lot of processed vegan foods, which are very high in wheat. I started developing severe joint pains and gained weight. It was towards the end of the two years that I was introduced to the Blood Type Diet. I discovered that my blood type actually does better with meat proteins and when we switched back to eating meats, I actually lost twelve pounds in the first week. It was at this time that it was also recommended that I cut gluten from my diet to see if it would help relieve any of the joint issues. To my surprise it did, which is the reason we also went gluten-free at about the same time.

## VEGETARIAN

A vegetarian is a person who does not eat meat, including poultry, game, fish, shellfish, or any animal derived products, such as gelatin. Vegetarians typically abstain from consuming animal-based foods for ethical, environmental, health, or other reasons. Some vegetarians may also abstain from using animal-derived products, such as leather, fur, or wool.

NOTES:_____

_____

Vegetarians may follow a plant-based diet, which includes a variety of grains, beans, vegetables, fruits, nuts, and seeds, or they may follow a more restricted diet that excludes certain foods, such as eggs or dairy products. Vegetarians may also follow a vegan diet, which excludes all animal-derived products, including eggs, dairy, and honey.

## WELL-BEING

Well-being refers to a state of physical, mental, and social well-being. It encompasses a person's overall health, happiness, and prosperity. In terms of the human body, well-being can refer to the absence of physical illness or injury, as well as the presence of physical fitness and vitality. It can also involve emotional and mental well-being, such as feeling happy, fulfilled, and at peace with oneself.

Social well-being, which is often connected to physical and emotional well-being, involves having supportive relationships, feeling connected to others, and participating in activities that bring meaning and purpose to one's life. Overall, well-being is a multifaceted concept that encompasses a wide range of factors that contribute to a person's overall health and happiness.

## WILLPOWER

Willpower is the mental or emotional strength that allows a person to persevere, resist temptation, and control their actions and behaviors. It is the ability to make conscious choices and decisions, especially when faced with challenges or obstacles, and to follow through on those choices despite any distractions or

NOTES:_____

_____

temptations that may arise. Willpower is often associated with determination, self-discipline, and self-control, and it is a crucial factor in achieving goals and overcoming obstacles. It requires effort and practice to develop and maintain, but it can be a powerful tool for personal growth and success.

These are just a few of the thousands of health related terms and this is just the beginning of your self-education about health and happiness. There are many online resources available to help you expand your knowledge even further, so feel free to explore what is out there.

Be sure that the information you access is from a reliable and reputable source, you don't want to become the victim of the blind leading the blind!

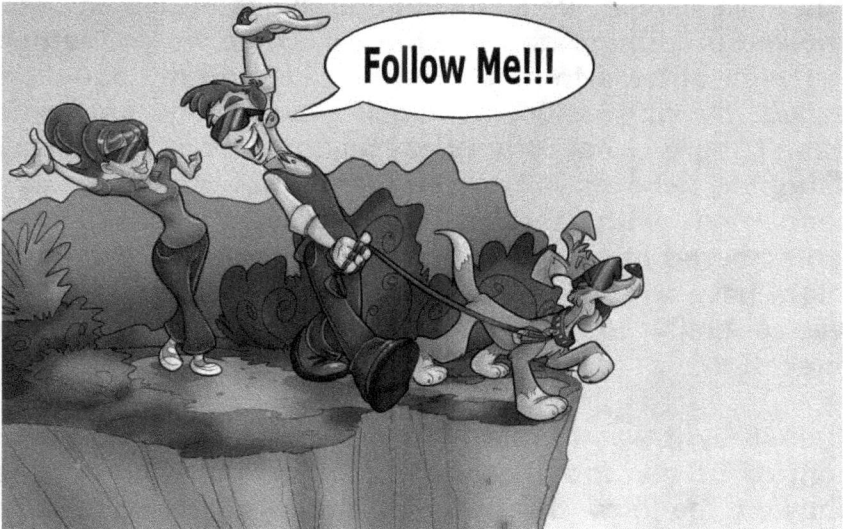

NOTES:_____

# AN UNEXPECTED TWIST

During the tail end of my recent health journey I discovered an interesting twist. It made me realize just how cynical the world has made people. It may be hard to believe, but I was inspired to write this book during a cross-country move from California to Florida during the final months of 2022. In fact, this book went from just an idea to being finished in less than four months.

We made the trip in our RV, stopping to see friends and family along the way. One of those stops was to visit my daughter and my grandkids in Missouri. It had been quite some time since we had seen each other, so her most recent personal memory of me was when I was much heavier.

When we arrived, we all exchanged pleasantries and she showed us around her new house. Once we got settled in I went outside to play with the kids and my daughter pulled my wife aside, asking if I was okay. My wife wasn't sure what she was talking about, until my daughter, who is a nurse, mentioned that she was concerned with the way I looked. She never remembered me ever looking so thin and she thought I might have a medical issue, like cancer, and that the trip was actually to say goodbyes instead of a simple relocation.

Thankfully it wasn't and I was thin because I had taken control of my food, eating habits and my life. This showed me how the state of the world can make a person immediately think a worst case scenario, instead of the possibility that someone had decided to make some drastic changes in order to see drastic results. Share your journey with others, so when they see the New You, they will know it is who you set out to be!

NOTES:_____

_____

## HEALTH AND HAPPINESS

When it comes to happiness, good health is kind of a gateway drug. Until you find good health, happiness may be very challenging to obtain. When you feel miserable, it is extremely difficult to be happy.

It is fair to say that good health is vital to finding happiness. Losing your health usually ends up creating a domino effect, with other aspects of life becoming more difficult to handle. I know for me, when my health was questionable, almost all aspects of my life were on the brink of ruin. Life felt like a continuous avalanche. Just day after day of feeling buried, smothered and trapped!

It's amazing how regaining or discovering good health for the first time can create a heatwave of hope that has the ability to melt away the snow of life's avalanches! Suddenly the days don't seem so bleak, you don't feel quite as buried, you can actually breathe a little. If you have experienced your own life avalanche, you're not alone and there can be peace and warmth at the end of the storm!

*YOU DESERVE TO BE HEALTHY*

*YOU DESERVE TO BE HAPPY*

NOTES:_____

_____

# IN CLOSING

I hope the lessons and insights shared within the pages of this book have helped you on your journey towards personal growth and self-improvement. Your dedication to bettering yourself is inspiring, and I'm honored to have been a part of that process.

Remember, growth is an ongoing process, and the tools and techniques shared in this book are just the beginning. Keep learning, keep growing, and continue to be the best version of yourself.

Life is a precious gift and it is important to make the most of it. But what is truly important in life? The answer is different for everyone, but there are a few things that are universally considered to be important in life.

One of the most important things in life is the ability to connect with others. Human beings are social creatures and we thrive on connection and relationships. Whether it is through family, friends, or romantic relationships, having a strong support system is vital for our well-being.

Achieving personal growth and self-awareness is also important in life. This means taking the time to reflect on our thoughts, feelings, and actions, and making changes to become the best version of ourselves.

Lastly, it is important to find balance and harmony in life. This means taking care of our physical, emotional, and mental well-being. It also means finding balance between work, leisure, and relationships.

NOTES:_____
_____

**Dear Reader,**

I hope this book, "New You", has been a meaningful and helpful journey for you on your path towards a healthier and happier life. It has been a privilege to be a part of your growth and I am grateful for the opportunity to be part of this journey.

Your decision to invest in yourself by reading this book is a testament to your determination and commitment to becoming a better version of yourself. I am confident that you have gained valuable insights and tools to help you achieve your goals and live a fulfilling life.

I want to express my sincere gratitude for choosing "New You" and for taking the time to read it. Your support and interest in my work means the world to me.

As you move forward, I wish you continued success and happiness in all aspects of your life. Remember that your health and well-being are your greatest assets and taking care of them should be a top priority.

I hope that you have found the information in this book to be empowering and inspiring. I trust that you will continue to make positive changes in your life and that you will continue to strive towards becoming the best version of yourself.

Once again, thank you for reading "New You". I hope that it has been a valuable and transformative experience for you.

Wishing you good health and true happiness,

231

NOTES:_____

_____

# NEW YOU PERSONAL GOAL SETTING

Remember the section on setting goals?  Well, the time has come for you to set your initial goals.  It is very important to set goals, so you know what you are working towards and how to get there.  A journey without a destination is called "wandering"!

Below are some suggested initial goals for you to set. Make sure that your goals are realistic and obtainable, otherwise they're not goals they're wishes and we're not here to make wishes, we're here to make the New You!

**CURRENT WEIGHT & DATE** _____

**30-DAY WEIGHT GOAL** _____

**30-DAY WEIGHT** _____

**60-DAY WEIGHT GOAL** _____

**60-DAY WEIGHT** _____

**90-DAY WEIGHT GOAL** _____

**90-DAY WEIGHT** _____

As a reminder, the reason I waited until now to have you set goals is because I wanted you to be empowered with information this book has to offer BEFORE setting your goals.  Why?  Because now you have some of the knowledge necessary to effectively pursue those goals. So now it's time to set your goals and use your new found knowledge to achieve them.

## *Welcome to your official New You journey!*

NOTES:_____

_____

www.ingramcontent.com/pod-product-compliance
Lightning Source LLC
Chambersburg PA
CBHW061015280326
41935CB00009B/974